Imaging of Airway Diseases

Guest Editor

PHILIPPE A. GRENIER, MD

RADIOLOGIC CLINICS
OF NORTH AMERICA

www.radiologic.theclinics.com

March 2009 • Volume 47 • Number 2

SAUNDERS an imprint of ELSEVIER, Inc.

W.B. SAUNDERS COMPANY
A Division of Elsevier Inc.

1600 John F. Kennedy Boulevard • Suite 1800 • Philadelphia, Pennsylvania 19103-2899

http://www.theclinics.com

RADIOLOGIC CLINICS OF NORTH AMERICA Volume 47, Number 2
March 2009 ISSN 0033-8389, ISBN 13: 978-1-4377-0536-2, ISBN 10: 1-4377-0536-7

Editor: Barton Dudlick
Developmental Editor: Theresa Collier

Radiologic Clinics of North America (ISSN 0033-8389) is published bimonthly in January, March, May, July, September, and November by Elsevier Inc., 360 Park Avenue South, New York, NY 10010-1710. Business and Editorial Offices: 1600 John F. Kennedy Boulevard., Suite 1800, Philadelphia, PA 19103-2899. Customer Service Office: 11830 Westline Industrial Drive, St. Louis, MO 63146. Periodicals postage paid at New York, NY and additional mailing offices. Subscription prices are USD 328 per year for US individuals, USD 487 per year for US institutions, USD 160 per year for US students and residents, USD 383 per year for Canadian individuals, USD 611 per year for Canadian institutions, USD 473 per year for international individuals, USD 611 per year for international institutions, and USD 230 per year for Canadian and foreign students/residents. To receive student and resident rate, orders must be accompanied by name of affiliated institution, date of term and the signature of program/residency coordinatior on institution letterhead. Orders will be billed at individual rate until proof of status is received. Foreign air speed delivery is included in all *Clinics* subscription prices. All prices are subject to change without notice. **POSTMASTER:** Send address changes to *Radiologic Clinics of North America*, Elsevier Journals Customer Service, 11830 Westline Industrial Drive, St. Louis, MO 63146. **Customer Service: 1-800-654-2452 (US and Canada). From outside of the United States and Canada, call 1-314-453-7041. Fax: 1-314-453-5170. E-mail: JournalsCustomerService-usa@elsevier.com (for print support) and JournalsOnlineSupport-usa@elsevier. com (for online support).**

Reprints. For copies of 100 or more of articles in this publication, please contact the Commercial Reprints Department, Elsevier Inc., 360 Park Avenue South, New York, New York 10010-1710. Tel.: (+1) 212-633-3812; Fax: (+1) 212-462-1935; E-mail: reprints@elsevier.com.

Radiologic Clinics of North America also published in Greek Paschalidis Medical Publications, Athens, Greece.

Radiologic Clinics of North America is covered in *MEDLINE/PubMed (Index Medicus), EMBASE/Excerpta Medica, Current Contents/Life Sciences, Current Contents/Clinical Medicine, RSNA Index to Imaging Literature, BIOSIS, Science Citation Index,* and *ISI/BIOMED.*

Printed and bound in the United Kingdom
Transferred to Digital Print 2011

Contributors

GUEST EDITOR

PHILIPPE A. GRENIER, MD
Professor of Radiology, Service de Radiologie
Polyvalente, Diagnostique et Interventionnelle,
Hôpital Pitié-Salpêtrière, Paris, France

AUTHORS

TSHERING AMDO, MD
Division of Pulmonary and Critical Care Medicine,
New York University-Langone Medical Center,
Tisch Hospital, New York, New York

F. ARBIB, MD
Consultant, Clinique de Pneumologie,
CHU Grenoble, France

CATHERINE BEIGELMAN-AUBRY, MD
Professor, College of Medicine, Hôpital
Pitié-Salpêtrière, Assistance Publique-Hôpitaux
de Paris (APHP), Université Pierre et Marie Curie
Service de Radiologie Polyvalente Diagnostique
et Interventionnelle, Paris, France

SANJEEV BHALLA, MD
Associate Professor of Radiology, Section of
Cardiothoracic Imaging, Mallinckrodt Institute
of Radiology, Washington University School
of Medicine, St. Louis, Missouri

C. BITHIGOFFER, MD
Université J Fourier, Clinique Universitaire de
Radiologie et Imagerie Médicale, CHU Grenoble,
France

PHILLIP M. BOISELLE, MD
Associate Professor, Department of Radiology,
Center for Airway Imaging, Beth Israel Deaconess
Medical Center, Harvard Medical School, Boston,
Massachusetts

PIERRE-YVES BRILLET, MD, PhD
Assistant Professor, Hôpital Avicenne, Assistance
Publique-Hôpitaux de Paris (APHP), Service de
Radiologie, Université Paris XIII, Bobigny, France

AMANDINE DESIR, MD
Resident in Radiology, Department of Medical
Imaging, University Hospital of Liège, Sart-Tilman,
Liège, Belgium

G.R. FERRETTI, MD, PhD
Professor of Radiology, Clinique Universitaire de
Radiologie et Imagerie Médicale, CHU Grenoble,
France; Université J Fourier, Grenoble, France;
and INSERM U 823, Institut A Bonniot, la Tronche,
France

BENOÎT GHAYE, MD
Chief of Clinics, Department of Medical Imaging,
University Hospital of Liège, Sart-Tilman, Liège,
Belgium

MYRNA C.B. GODOY, MD
Department of Radiology, New York
University-Langone Medical Center, Tisch
Hospital, New York, New York

PHILIPPE A. GRENIER, MD
Professor of Radiology, Hôpital Pitié-Salpêtrière,
Assistance Publique-Hôpitaux de Paris (APHP),
Université Pierre et Marie Curie Service de
Radiologie Polyvalente Diagnostique et
Interventionnelle, Paris, France

A. JANKOWSKI, MD
Université J Fourier, Clinique Universitaire de Radiologie et Imagerie Médicale, CHU Grenoble, France

CYLEN JAVIDAN-NEJAD, MD
Assistant Professor of Radiology, Section of Cardiothoracic Imaging, Mallinckrodt Institute of Radiology, Washington University School of Medicine, St. Louis, Missouri

HANS-ULRICH KAUCZOR, MD, PhD
Department of Pediatric Radiology; and Department of Diagnostic and Interventional Radiology, University Hospital Heidelberg, Heidelberg, Germany

S. LANTUEJOUL, MD, PhD
Professor of Pathology, Département d'Anatomie et Cytologie Pathologiques, CHU Grenoble, France; Université J Fourier, Grenoble, France; and INSERM U 823, Institut A Bonniot, la Tronche, France

EDWARD Y. LEE, MD, MPH
Assistant Professor, Departments of Radiology and Medicine, Pulmonary Division, Children's Hospital Boston, Harvard Medical School, Boston, Massachusetts

JULIA LEY-ZAPOROZHAN, MD
Department of Pediatric Radiology; and Department of Diagnostic and Interventional Radiology, University Hospital Heidelberg, Heidelberg, Germany

DIANA LITMANOVICH, MD
Instructor of Radiology, Department of Radiology, Center for Airway Imaging, Beth Israel Deaconess Medical Center, Harvard Medical School, Boston, Massachusetts

DAVID A. LYNCH, MB
Professor and Co-Director, Division of Radiology, National Jewish Health, Denver, Colorado

DAVID P. NAIDICH, MD, FACCP
Department of Radiology, New York University-Langone Medical Center, Tisch Hospital, New York, New York

DAVID OST, MD, MPH
Division of Pulmonary and Critical Care Medicine, New York University-Langone Medical Center, Tisch Hospital, New York, New York; and Division of Pulmonary Medicine, MD Anderson Cancer Center, Houston, Texas

SUDHAKAR N.J. PIPAVATH, MBBS
Department of Radiology, University of Washington Medical Center, Seattle, Washington

C.A. RIGHINI, MD, PhD
Assistant Professor of ENT, Université J Fourier, Clinique Universitaire de'ORL, CHU Grenoble, France; and INSERM U 823, Institut A Bonniot, la Tronche, France

ERIC J. STERN, MD
Professor, Department of Radiology, University of Washington Medical Center, Seattle, Washington

ALYN Q. WOODS, MD
Radiology Fellow, National Jewish Health, Denver, Colorado; and University of Colorado Denver Health Sciences Center, Radiology Academic Office, Aurora, Colorado

Contents

The new generation of multidetector CT (MDCT) has revolutionized noninvasive imaging of proximal and distal airways. Exquisite anatomic details of the airway lumen and airway wall on axial CT images benefit in routine practice from postprocessing tools in adequate orientation. This method ensures an excellent assessment of the morphology and location of any pathology. It may be combined with use of very low dose CT. Airway lumen and airway wall areas may be quantitatively assessed on MDCT images by using specific techniques that are reproducible and accurate.

Multidetector CT has broadened the potential of imaging to demonstrate anomalies of the lung and the tracheobronchial tree with increasing frequency. Two-and three-dimensional reformatting improve the understanding of complex tracheobronchial anomalies. Most congenital tracheobronchial anomalies are rare and almost always nonsymptomatic; however, some may be confused with or even responsible for respiratory disease. Tracheal and accessory cardiac bronchi are among the most frequent anomalies, but other ectopic or supernumerary lung buds, developmental tracheobronchial interruption, obstruction, or compression, communicating bronchopulmonary foregut malformations, and bronchial malformations associated with anomalies of situs can be detected, even late after birth.

Tumors of the trachea and central bronchi can be benign or malignant. Clinical presentation may be confusing, particularly in benign tumors that can be misdiagnosed as asthma or chronic bronchitis. Chest radiography has many limitations and is often considered unremarkable in patients with tumors of the central airways; therefore, multidetector CT (MDCT) has become the most useful noninvasive method for diagnosing and assessing the central airways. The purpose of this article is to provide a review of imaging of the tumors of the trachea and central bronchi. We emphasize the crucial role of MDCT and postprocessing techniques in assessing neoplasms of the central airways.

Nonneoplastic stenosis of proximal airways may result from longstanding intubations or tracheostomy, granulomatous infection, or systemic diseases such as relapsing polychondritis, amyloidosis, Wegener's granulomatosis, sarcoidosis, and inflammatory bowel disease. It also may be caused by saber sheath trachea, tracheobronchopathia osteoplastica, or broncholithiasis. An early diagnosis of the tracheal and bronchial stenosis has become possible with the advent of routine CT imaging. Multiplanar and volume rendering reformations after thin collimation MDCT acquisition help assess the location and extent of the stenosis and characterize the presence, distribution, and type of airway wall thickening. They also help surgeons and endoscopists to select adequate procedures and assess the response to treatment.

Tracheobronchomalacia (TBM) refers to excessive expiratory collapse of the trachea and bronchi as a result of weakening of the airway walls and/or supporting cartilage. This disorder has recently been increasingly recognized as an important cause of chronic respiratory symptoms. Multidetector CT (MDCT) technology allows for noninvasive imaging of TBM with similar accuracy to the historical reference standard of bronchoscopy. Paired end-inspiratory, dynamic expiratory MDCT is the examination of choice for assessing patients with suspected TBM. Radiologists should become familiar with imaging protocols and interpretation techniques to accurately diagnose this condition using MDCT.

The development and rapid advancement of both bronchoscopic, CT and ultrasound imaging technology has had considerable impact on the management of a wide variety of pulmonary diseases. The synergy between these newer imaging modalities and advanced interventional endoscopic procedures has led to a revolution in diagnostic and therapeutic options in patients with both central and peripheral airway disease. Given the broad clinical implications of these technological advances, only the most important areas of interventional pulmonology in which imaging has had a major impact will be selectively reviewed to highlight fundamental principles.

Bronchiectasis is defined as irreversible bronchial dilatation, leading to chronic cough, sputum formation, and recurrent infections. HRCT plays a major role in diagnosis of bronchiectasis. Most bronchiectasis is either idiopathic or a result of prior infections. Cystic fibrosis, allergic bronchopulmonary aspergillosis, and traction bronchiectasis caused by prior tuberculosis, sarcoidosis, and silicosis with progressive massive fibrosis have an upper lobe distribution. A lower lobe distribution is mostly seen in chronic aspiration, hypogammaglobulinemia, Mounier-Kuhn syndrome, primary ciliary dyskinesia, and traction bronchiectasis caused by usual interstitial pneumonitis and nonspecific interstitial pneumonitis. The right middle lobe and lingula are preferentially involved in atypical mycobacterial infections and sometimes in primary ciliary dyskinesia and Kartagener syndrome. A location-based approach may help lead to a specific diagnosis.

Radiologic Clinics of North America

THE CLINICS ARE NOW AVAILABLE ONLINE!

Access your subscription at:
www.theclinics.com

GOAL STATEMENT

The goal of the *Radiologic Clinics of North America* is to keep practicing radiologists and radiology residents up to date with current clinical practice in radiology by providing timely articles reviewing the state of the art in patient care.

ACCREDITATION

The *Radiologic Clinics of North America* is planned and implemented in accordance with the Essential Areas and Policies of the Accreditation Council for Continuing Medical Education (ACCME) through the joint sponsorship of the University of Virginia School of Medicine and Elsevier. The University of Virginia School of Medicine is accredited by the ACCME to provide continuing medical education for physicians.

The University of Virginia School of Medicine designates this educational activity for a maximum of 15 *AMA PRA Category 1 Credits*™. Physicians should only claim credit commensurate with the extent of their participation in the activity.

The American Medical Association has determined that physicians not licensed in the US who participate in this CME activity are eligible for 15 *AMA PRA Category 1 Credits*™.

Credit can be earned by reading the text material, taking the CME examination online at http://www.theclinics.com/home/cme, and completing the evaluation. After taking the test, you will be required to review any and all incorrect answers. Following completion of the test and evaluation, your credit will be awarded and you may print your certificate.

FACULTY DISCLOSURE/CONFLICT OF INTEREST

The University of Virginia School of Medicine, as an ACCME accredited provider, endorses and strives to comply with the Accreditation Council for Continuing Medical Education (ACCME) Standards of Commercial Support, Commonwealth of Virginia statutes, University of Virginia policies and procedures, and associated federal and private regulations and guidelines on the need for disclosure and monitoring of proprietary and financial interests that may affect the scientific integrity and balance of content delivered in continuing medical education activities under our auspices.

The University of Virginia School of Medicine requires that all CME activities accredited through this institution be developed independently and be scientifically rigorous, balanced and objective in the presentation/discussion of its content, theories and practices.

All authors/editors participating in an accredited CME activity are expected to disclose to the readers relevant financial relationships with commercial entities occurring within the past 12 months (such as grants or research support, employee, consultant, stock holder, member of speakers bureau, etc.). The University of Virginia School of Medicine will employ appropriate mechanisms to resolve potential conflicts of interest to maintain the standards of fair and balanced education to the reader. Questions about specific strategies can be directed to the Office of Continuing Medical Education, University of Virginia School of Medicine, Charlottesville, Virginia.

The faculty and staff of the University of Virginia Office of Continuing Medical Education have no financial affiliations to disclose.

The authors/editors listed below have identified no financial or professional relationships for themselves or their spouse/partner:
Tshering Dorjee Amdo, MD; François Arbib, MD; Catherine Beigelman-Aubry, MD; Sanjeev Bhalla, MD; Christine Bithogoffer, MD; Philippe M. Boiselle, MD; Pierre-Yves Brillet, MD, PhD; Amandine Desir, MD; Barton Dudlick (Acquisitions Editor); Gilbert R. Ferretti, MD, PhD; Benoît Ghaye, MD; Myrna Cobos Barco Godoy, MD; Philippe A. Grenier, MD (Guest Editor); Aiden Jankowski, MD; Clyen Javidan-Nejad, MD; Hans-Ulrich Kauczor, MD, PhD; Theodore E. Keats, MD (Test Author); Sylvie Lantuejoul, MD, PhD; Edward Y. Lee, MD, MPH; Julia Ley-Zaporozhan, MD; Diana Litmanovich, MD; Christtian Adrien Righini, MD, PhD; Eric J. Stern, MD; and Alyn Q. Woods, MD.

The authors/editors listed below have identified the following financial or professional relationships for themselves or their spouse/partner:
David A. Lynch, MB is a consultant for Intermune, Inc., Gilead, Inc., and Centocor, Inc., and serves on the Advisory Board for Actelion, Inc.
David P. Naidich, MD, FACCP is a consultant and serves on the Advisory Board for Spiration.
David Ost, MD, MPH was part of a clinical trial with Broncus Technologies that involved no direct financial reimbursement.
Sudhakar N.J. Pipavath, MBBS owns stock in Reddy Labs.

Disclosure of Discussion of Non-FDA Approved Uses for Pharmaceutical Products and/or Medical Devices.

The University of Virginia School of Medicine, as an ACCME provider, requires that all faculty presenters identify and disclose any off-label uses for pharmaceutical and medical device products. The University of Virginia School of Medicine recommends that each physician fully review all the available data on new products or procedures prior to clinical use.

TO ENROLL

To enroll in the Radiologic Clinics of North America Continuing Medical Education program, call customer service at 1-800-654-2452 or sign up online at http://www.theclinics.com/home/cme. The CME program is available to subscribers for an additional annual fee USD 205.

Preface

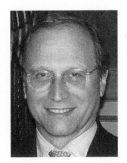

Philippe A. Grenier, MD
Guest Editor

In the past 20 years, remarkable technologic advances in CT imaging have revolutionized noninvasive imaging of all thoracic structures, including the airways. CT has assumed a central position in the modern management of both focal and diffuse airway diseases. The combination of thin collimation and helical acquisition during a single breath-hold at full inspiration multidetector CT (MDCT) provides high-resolution volumetric data sets that allow the generation of high-quality multiplanar and three-dimensional images of the airways. Accurate assessment and anatomical display of proximal and distal airways are routinely obtained. In addition, dynamic acquisition during a forced expiratory maneuver is highly appreciated to detect and assess obstruction on small airways and abnormal collapse of large airways.

Nowadays, MDCT is used not only to detect neoplastic and non-neoplastic endotracheal and endobronchial lesions and to assess the extent of tracheobronchial stenosis for planning treatment and follow-up, but also to diagnose and assess the extent of bronchiectasis and small-airway disease, and, in addition, to detect bronchial fistula, cysts, or dehiscences.

In parallel, there have also been important advances in diagnostic and interventional bronchoscopy and surgery. In this respect, the information provided by CT has become increasingly essential for establishing accurate diagnoses, for guiding and planning procedures, and for assessing response to therapy. Recent improvement in image analysis techniques has made possible accurate and reproducible quantitative analysis of airway wall and lumen areas, as well as lung volume and attenuation, leading to better insights in physiopathology of obstructive lung disease, particularly chronic obstructive pulmonary disease and asthma.

The authors of this issue of *Radiologic Clinics of North America* were chosen for their focused expertise in airway imaging. I thank those chest radiologists for sharing their experience and insights to provide a comprehensive update on practical imaging for airway disease. While high-resolution CT and MDCT have tremendously improved our ability to assess large- and small-airway diseases, I anticipate even more developments in the future. Rapid-volume scanning and new postprocessing techniques may promote sophisticated functional imaging and advanced interventions. MR imaging in this respect may become an additional modality to MDCT.

Philippe A. Grenier, MD
Service de Radiologie Polyvalente
Diagnostique et Interventionnelle
Hopital Pitie-Salpetriere
47-83, boulevard de l'Hopital
75651 Paris cedex 13, France

E-mail address:
philippe.grenier@psl.aphp.fr (P.A. Grenier)

Radiol Clin N Am 47 (2009) xi
doi:10.1016/j.rcl.2009.01.007

MDCT of the Airways: Technique and Normal Results

Catherine Beigelman-Aubry, MD[a], Pierre-Yves Brillet, MD, PhD[b],
Philippe A. Grenier, MD[a],*

KEYWORDS
• Trachea anatomy • Bronchi anatomy
• Airway dimensions • Airway MDCT technique

Previously, the trachea and main bronchi were assessed with a variable slice thickness up to 5 mm with sequential or volumetric CT, and small airways diseases were explored with high-resolution CT (HRCT), based on a 1.5-mm slice at 10-mm intervals. Currently, the new generation of multidetector CT (MDCT) by combining volumetric CT acquisition and thin collimation during a single breathhold provides an accurate continuous assessment from the trachea to the most distal airway visible. Isotropic voxels allow image reconstructions in which the z dimension is equivalent to the x and y (in plane) resolution.[1] This approach creates multiplanar reformations of high quality along the long axis of the airways[2] and three-dimensional volume rendering, including extraction of the airway and virtual endoscopy without any distortion in any orientation. Whatever their nature and severity, excellent assessments of stenoses may be obtained by a combination of various reconstructions, especially the determination of the morphology, including the identification of horizontal webs and the length and exact location from the vocal cords and carina.[3,4] Airway stents and extrinsic airway compression are also assessed perfectly. Preprocedural planning before stent placement or surgery[3] and posttherapeutic aspects also benefit from the same techniques. Despite images usually being obtained during suspended inspiration for analysis of airways, a complementary acquisition during forced expiratory maneuver may be requested to assess the degree of tracheobronchomalacia and the extent of air trapping.

IMAGE ACQUISITION AND RECONSTRUCTION

Because the lung parenchyma offers a unique natural contrast, low radiation dose may be used without significant loss of information (100–120 kV, 60–160 mAs). Using a detector size of 0.625 mm with MDCT, images are reconstructed with a slice thickness of approximately 1 mm and overlapped with a reconstruction interval of approximately one-half slice thickness. This produces a resolution voxel of almost cubic dimensions of approximately 0.4 mm in each direction by using a spatial resolution algorithm. Experts recommend using a 512 or even a 768 matrix, which permits fields of view of 265 mm and 400 mm, respectively. The pixel size at the workstation, which is defined as the ratio between the field of view and the matrix, has to be lower than the intrinsic resolution in the plane of image to benefit from the intrinsic resolution capabilities of the equipment.[5]

A rotation time of approximately 500 msec allows an important decrease in cardiac pulsation artifacts and allows a good analysis of all bronchi, including the paracardiac areas. Breathholding for acquisition of the entire chest lasts approximately 6 to 8 seconds using a 40 or 64 detector row CT scanner, which avoids respiratory motion artifacts

[a] Service de Radiologie, Hôpital Pitié-Salpêtrière, Assistance Publique-Hôpitaux de Paris (APHP), Université Pierre et Marie Curie, 47/83 boulevard de l'Hôpital, 75651 Paris cedex 13, France
[b] Service de Radiologie, Hôpital Avicenne, Assistance Publique-Hôpitaux de Paris (APHP), Université Paris XIII, UPRES EA 2363, Hôpital Avicenne, 125, route de Stalingrad, 93009 Bobigny, France
* Corresponding author.
E-mail address: philippe.grenier@psl.aphp.fr (P.A. Grenier).

Radiol Clin N Am 47 (2009) 185–201
doi:10.1016/j.rcl.2009.01.001

in most cases. The use of cardiac gating is not recommended because of the higher radiation dose delivered and short rotation time available with the last generations of MDCT.

READING AND POSTPROCESSING TOOLS
Cine Viewing

Visualization of overlapped thin axial images sequentially in a cine mode allows analysis of bronchial divisions from the segmental origin down to the smallest bronchi that can be identified on thin section images. Particular attention must be paid to the analysis of the lumen of the tracheobronchial tree, the airway walls, and the spurs at the same time. Moving up and down through the volume at the monitor has become a useful alternative to film-based review. This viewing technique helps indicate the exact location of any airway lesion and may serve as a roadmap for the endoscopist. Reading of chest MDCT goes actually far beyond the standard assessment of axial slices, because multiplanar reformats are easily performed in real time in all directions[6] and slabs with various rendering modes. Once any abnormality has been detected, an oblique reformat plane may be chosen with the swivel mode by focusing a rotation center on the abnormality

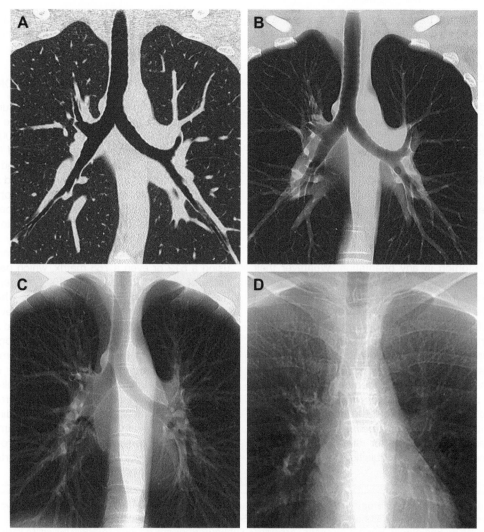

Fig. 1. (*A*) Down and backward 1.41-mm oblique reformat allows visualization of the trachea, carina, main bronchi, and some segmental and subsegmental bronchi. Progressive thickening of the slabs—17 mm (*B*) and 54 mm (*C*)—allows reproduction of previous tomographic aspects with better understanding of the underlying pathology, especially for the airways. (*D*) Slab average of 180 mm thickness allows reproduction of the aspect of the frontal chest radiograph. The right tracheal stripe is clearly explained by the correlation on (*A*).

found. A combination of slabs of various thicknesses with minimum intensity projection (mIP) or maximum intensity projection (MIP) or both usually is obtained.

Two-Dimensional Reformats and Multiplanar Volume Rendering Slabs

Reformations and reconstructions are easy to generate and may be interactively performed in real-time at the console or workstation. Multiplanar reformation images are single-voxel sections with a 0.6- to 0.8-mm displayed image. They are the easiest reconstructions to generate and permit creation of images oriented in any plane, especially along the long axis of any airway (eg, in a coronal oblique orientation for the trachea and the carina). On the other hand, multiplanar volume reformation consists of a slab of adjacent thin slices of various thicknesses that may be combined with the use of intensity projection techniques. The reformation plane may be selected by focusing a rotation center on the abnormality and using the swivel mode or using a three-dimensional reconstructed image of the airways.[7] A significant decrease in the number of slices to be analyzed is achieved by analysis of longitudinal reformats compared with the axial images with a complementary role of both viewing techniques.

Analysis of various large and small airway diseases may be enhanced with this technique. In fact, multiplanar volume reformation images combine the excellent spatial resolution of multiplanar reformats images with the anatomic display of thick slices[8] and the possibility of using various rendering tools:

- Average: the mean attenuation value of the voxels in every view throughout the volume explored is projected on a two-dimensional image. A less noisy image may be obtained de facto. Tomographic equivalent images may be obtained by thickening the slabs with equivalent of plain films in the coronal and lateral views with the thickest slabs (Fig. 1).
- mIP imaging is a simple form of volume rendering (sliding thin slab or multiplanar volume reformation mIP technique) that is able to project the tracheobronchial air column onto a viewing plane by projecting the pixels with the lowest attenuation value. This technique enhances the visibility of the airways within lung parenchyma below the subsubsegmental level because of lower attenuation of air contained within the tracheobronchial tree compared with the

surrounding pulmonary parenchyma (Fig. 2), with a difference of density between 50 and 150 HU.[9] The overall morphology of the tracheobronchial tree is particularly well displayed on longitudinal views combined with a multiplanar volume reformation mIP technique. Three- to 7-mm slabs are particularly adapted for the assessment of central airways stenosis, but the slab thickness may be chosen according to the complexity and morphology of the abnormality and may be increased up to several centimeters. Abnormal lucencies, including bronchial wall diverticula observed in patients who have chronic obstructive pulmonary disease and bronchial anastomosis, dehiscence, or fistula during or after lung transplantation, may be assessed using the same technique. Multiplanar volume reformation mIP is also used for a systematic analysis of the parietal wall and lumen of the bronchi. This analysis also includes the assessment of peribronchial thickening encountered in case of lung diseases with a perilymphatic distribution. In chronic bronchial disease, bronchial wall thickening is often irregular and associated with thickening of the spurs and irregularities in the morphology and caliber of the bronchi. This technique may help plan the correct bronchoscopic pathway toward a distal lesion for biopsy. Postexpiratory mIP

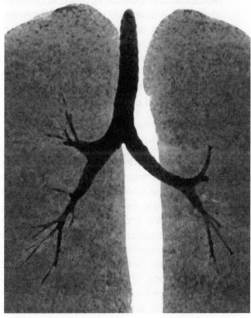

Fig. 2. Coronal mIP 60-mm slab allows display of the normal bronchial tree to the subsegmental level.

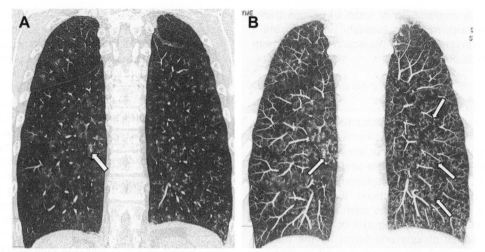

Fig. 3. Single (A) and 14-mm slab MIP (B) coronal reformats in a patient suffering from infectious bronchiolitis. (A) Patchy ground-glass bronchoalveolar nodules with bronchial wall thickening (*white arrow*). (B) Diffuse tree in bud aspects (*black and white arrows*) difficult to assess in (A) are obvious with MIP.

images may be useful for detecting and assessing the extent of air trapping.

- MIP consists of projecting the voxel with the highest attenuation value in every view through the volume explored.[10,11] It displays 10% of the data set, as does the mIP technique. Centrilobular nodules related to inflammatory or infectious changes in the small airways are easily recognized with respect to landmarks of the secondary pulmonary lobule (Fig. 3).[12] A rapid assessment of the regional distribution in the craniocaudal and axial dimensions is obtained at the same time. MIP of variable thickness also provides an excellent assessment of the location and size of vessels. In this way, mosaic perfusion pattern is diagnosed by combination of mIP and MIP and is easily differentiated from mosaic attenuation pattern caused by infiltrative lung disease.

External Three-Dimensional Rendering Technique

The volume-rendering technique applied at the level of the airways ensures a three-dimensional reconstruction of the airways to the subsegmental level by depicting the inner surface of the airway with a specific color and opacity (Fig. 4). It has capabilities of visualization in semi-transparent mode similar to conventional bronchograms.[13] For this reason, this technique has been referred as CT bronchography. Three-dimensional segmentation techniques provide an anatomic map of the airways and easily may demonstrate changes between inspiration and expiration in the case of tracheomalacia.

This technique has proved to be of particular interest in diagnosing mild changes in airway caliber and understanding complex tracheobronchial abnormalities.[14] When correlating bronchoscopy and three-dimensional reconstructions, Kauczor and colleagues[15] observed no

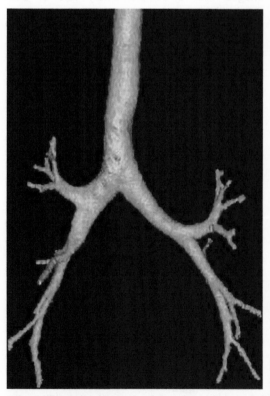

Fig. 4. Three-dimensional volume rendering of a normal tracheobronchial tree.

discrepancies concerning the location and severity of central stenoses. Three-dimensional helical CT provided an accurate road map for the central airways. Clinical relevance in patients with tumors resulted from severe stenoses or occlusions that lead to dyspnea and stridor. When bronchoscopy revealed severe stenosis or total occlusion, the patency of distal bronchi, tumor involvement, or collapse could not be assessed bronchoscopically. In comparison, three-dimensional helical CT was superior at showing the residual lumen and length of the stenoses, spatial orientation, branching angles, and patency of distal air-filled bronchi. These complementary details were important for possible endobronchial procedures such as laser ablation, stent placement, and transbronchial radiotherapy. This approach facilitated the choice of endobronchial procedures, and the size of the stent could be determined accurately.

Using the same concept, Fetita and colleagues[16] developed a fully automatic method for three-dimensional reconstruction of the tracheobronchial tree based on bronchial lumen detection within the thoracic volume data set obtained from thin MDCT acquisition. It provides a specific visualization modality that relies on energy-based three-dimensional reconstruction of the bronchial tree up to the sixth or seventh order subdivisions with a semi-transparent volume rendering technique.[17] Automatic delimitation and indexation of anatomic segments make local and reproducible analysis possible at any level of the bronchial tree. Automatic extraction of the central axis of the bronchial tree allows interactivity during navigation within CT bronchography or virtual endoscopy modes.

Internal Rendering Technique or Virtual Bronchoscopy

Virtual bronchoscopy by combining helical CT data and virtual reality computing techniques[13]

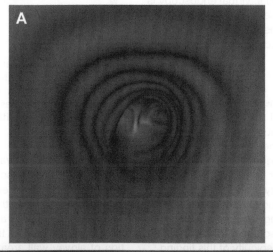

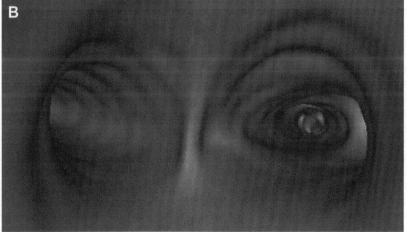

Fig. 5. Virtual endoscopy at the level of the middle trachea (*A*) and the carina (*B*).

provides an internal rendering of the tracheobronchial walls and lumen by using reconstruction with soft kernel. An endoscopist's view of the internal surface of the airways is simulated with a perspective-rendering algorithm (Fig. 5). The observer may interactively move through the airway at a rate of 15 to 25 images/second down to the subsegmental bronchi. Potential applications include the assessment of airway stenoses and guidance of transbronchial biopsy procedures.[18] The technique allows accurate reproduction of major endoluminal abnormalities and has excellent correlation with fiberoptic bronchoscopy results regarding the location, shape, and severity of airway narrowing. Virtual bronchoscopy is also able to evaluate the airways distal to a high-grade stenosis, beyond which a conventional bronchoscope cannot pass.[19] It is also possible to perform retroscopy when looking back toward the distal part of the stenosis. Virtual endoscopy may be considered a substitute for repeated bronchoscopies when performed in the follow-up of interventional procedures.[20] Despite its potential, virtual endoscopy is unable to identify the causes of bronchial obstruction[21] or detect mild stenosis, submucosal infiltration, and superficial spreading tumors.[4]

LEVEL OF BREATHING

All CT examinations of the airways are first performed at suspended full inspiration. In case of suspicion of mosaic attenuation or bronchomalacia, expiration has to be performed on a dynamic mode. In fact, this technique has proved to optimize the detection of air trapping, which is an indirect sign of small airway disease,[22] and tracheobronchomalacia.[23] The advantage of volumetric acquisition in this setting is use of mIP that enhances the visual detectability of air trapping and may increase the conspicuity of this finding,[24] even using low-dose CT (Fig. 6).[25]

QUANTITATIVE CT ASSESSMENT OF AIRWAYS

Airway lumen and airway wall areas may be assessed quantitatively on CT images by using specific techniques that must be reproducible and accurate to compare the airways before and after therapy and carry out longitudinal studies of airway remodeling. Because airway lumen and wall areas measured on axial images depend on lung volume, volumetric acquisition at controlled lung volume is required to precisely match the airways of an individual on repeated studies. Lumen and wall areas measured on axial images also depend on the angle between the airway central axis and the plane of section. Measuring

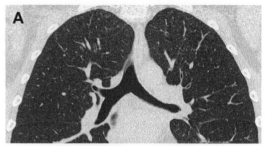
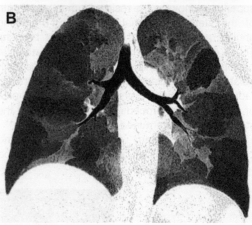

Fig. 6. Patient suffering relapsing polychondritis. (A) Normal aspect on inspiration is visualized on a volume from the vocal cords to the lower pulmonary veins. (B) Multifocal air trapping is assessed on 20-mm slab coronal mIP reformat despite the fact that the acquisition was performed with only 15 mAs.

airway lumen and airway walls when they are not perpendicular to the scanning plane may lead to significant errors related to an overestimation of airway wall area, as in the case of oblique bronchi. The larger the angle and field of view and the thicker the collimation, the greater the overestimation of airway wall area. Accurate measurements of airway lumen and wall area have to be restricted to airways that appear rounded (ie, cut in cross-section). The new generation of multislice CT scanner allows segmentation of bronchial lumens with three-dimensional reconstruction of the airways, extraction of the central axis of the airways, and reconstruction of the airway cross-section in a plane perpendicular to this axis (Fig. 7).[26]

Numerous techniques have been reported for measuring airway diameter using CT. They have been validated using data from phantom studies and excised animal lungs or by developing realistic modeling of airways and pulmonary arteries included in CT scans of animal lungs obtained in vivo.[27–32] These techniques have proved to be more accurate than those obtained with manual

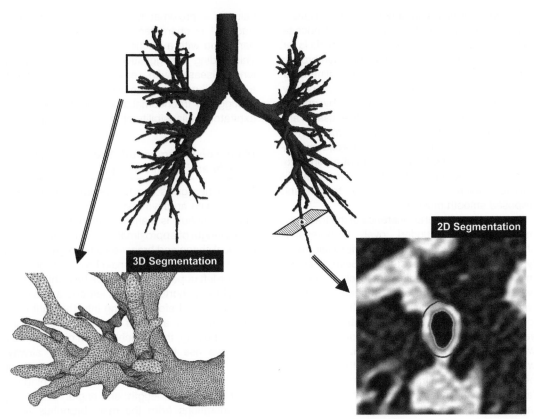

Fig. 7. Segmentation of bronchial lumens with three-dimensional reconstruction of the airways, extraction of the central axis of the airways, and reconstruction of a subsegmental branch of the posterior basal segmental bronchus of the left lower lobe (LLL) cross-section in a plane perpendicular to this axis.

methods. In fact, manual tracing of the inner and outer contours of the airway cross-section on axial CT images is a time-consuming technique that suffers from large intra- and interobserver variability in measurement of airway wall and lumen areas.[29,33–35] Their accuracy in measuring the airway lumen[27–29,31] and wall[28,30] areas was good only for bronchi that measured at least 2 mm in diameter. These techniques have been used to quantify the magnitude and distribution of airway narrowing in excised lung animals and animal lungs in vivo and in normal patients and patients who have asthma.[27,29,36–38] Although the techniques have been used almost exclusively for research purposes, with continued refinements they eventually will be beneficial in the clinical practice of radiology.[39–41]

NORMAL ANATOMY AND NORMAL CT FINDINGS
Trachea

The conducting airways that distribute air to the gas-exchanging units begin with the trachea. The trachea, which originates at the inferior margin of the cricoid cartilage at the level of the sixth cervical vertebra to the carina at the level of the fifth thoracic vertebra, has an oblique course downwards and backwards. Its length on inspiration has a value of 10 to 12 cm in adults, including the extrathoracic (2–4 cm) and intrathoracic portions (6–9 cm).[42,43] Changes in position may be observed between inspiration and expiration,[44] up to 3 cm, and with neck flexion and extension.

Adjacent structures directly related to the trachea are the thyroid gland, which is anterior and lateral to the cervical trachea, vessels anterior to the intrathoracic trachea (supra-aortic vessels, aortic arch, pulmonary arteries), systemic veins (superior vena cava, azygos vein), which are anterolateral or lateral to the trachea, lymph nodes, the esophagus, which is posterior or lateral to the trachea, and the left recurrent nerve. The trachea is often displaced slightly to the right at the level of the aortic arch, which may be accentuated in older patients with tortuous atherosclerotic aorta. The right or posterior tracheal wall contacts the right lung at a variable extent.[42]

The tracheal wall is comprised of several layers, including an inner mucosa layer, a submucosa, cartilage or muscle, and an outer adventicia layer. The anterior walls of the trachea and main bronchi are formed with U-shaped rings of hyaline cartilage—16 to 22 for the trachea—that open dorsally. These rings are linked longitudinally by annular ligaments of fibrous and connective tissue and help support the tracheal wall and maintain an adequate tracheal lumen during forced expiration.[43] The flat dorsal wall consists of a thin fibromuscular membrane that includes the trachealis muscle, which is composed by transversely disposed smooth muscle.[45]

The cross-sectional appearance of the trachea is most commonly rounded, oval, or horseshoe shape on inspiration, with a posterior wall that is typically flat or convex posteriorly. Several shapes may be encountered at different levels.[42] The right wall of the inferior aspect of the trachea is in contact with air within the medial aspect of the right upper lobe, which results in the right paratracheal stripe seen in routine posteroanterior chest radiographs with a normal size less than 4 mm. The tracheal wall appears as a 1- to 3-mm soft-tissue stripe between the air-filled tracheal lumen and the lateral fat density of the mediastinum.[42,46,47] Normal cartilaginous rings may appear slightly denser than surrounding soft tissue and fat. Calcification of the cartilage is commonly seen in older patients, particularly women, at the level of the trachea and more distal bronchi (Fig. 8). These calcifications are usually discontinuous.[42]

The normal transverse diameter of the trachea in men and women is 13 to 25 mm and 10 to 21 mm, respectively, and the normal anteroposterior diameter in men and women is 13 to 27 mm and 10 to 23 mm, respectively. The tracheal diameter averages 19.5 mm in men and 17.5 mm in women.[43,46,48] A mean decrease in the transverse diameter of approximately 15%, in the anteroposterior diameter of approximately 30%, and in the cross-sectional area of the trachea of approximately 35% is observed on forced expiration, mainly related to invagination of the posterior tracheal membrane. On expiration, the posterior tracheal membrane appears convex anteriorly; the horseshoe shape ensures actual patient expiration. Tracheomegaly is defined in men as a tracheal diameter of more than 25 mm in the transverse diameter and more than 27 mm in the anteroposterior dimension. In women it is defined as tracheal diameter of more than 21 mm in the transverse diameter and more than 23 mm in the anteroposterior dimension.[49]

The tracheal index is obtained by dividing the coronal diameter by the sagittal one, with a normal value of approximately 1.[42,43,47] A "saber sheath trachea" is characterized by a marked coronal narrowing with a tracheal index of less than 0.5. This finding is suggestive of chronic obstructive lung disease with emphysema. Conversely, a "lunate" configuration with a ratio of more than 1 suggests tracheomalacia related to excessive expiratory collapsibility of the airway lumen.[50]

Main, Lobar, Segmental, Subsegmental Bronchi and Small Airways

The trachea gives rise to the right and left main bronchi with an asymmetrical branching. The left main bronchus is narrower than the right one, with a length of approximately 5 cm[51] and a typical elliptical shape and branches off at a greater angle than the right.[52] The left main bronchus branches into the left upper and lower lobe bronchi. The right bronchus is shorter than the left one and extends for 1 to 2 cm before dividing into the right upper lobe bronchus and the bronchus intermedius. Within the lung, the bronchi branch dichotomously and give rise to progressively smaller airways. Branching is asymmetrical, taking into account that the two daughters of a given branching may differ in diameter, length, and angle. The number of generations from the main bronchus to the acini varies from as few as 8 to as many as 25, depending on the region of the lung supplied.[52] The lobar bronchi branch off to segmental bronchi.

Several systems for labeling segmental anatomy have been proposed, mainly the Jackson and Huber and the Boyden classifications.[53,54] Segmental bronchi are designated by "B" followed by a number, and subsegmental bronchi are indicated by the segmental number followed by a lower case letter. The numbering of the segmental bronchi corresponds to their order of origin from the airway. Although the segmental bronchial anatomy varies, the right lung contains ten segmental bronchi and the left contains eight in most patients. The first Boyden classification, which initially designated the anterior segment as B2 and the posterior segment as B3, is used in this article (Figs. 9–12). Identification of the origin of most bronchi depends on recognizing the spurs that separate them. Depending on its angle relative to the CT plane, a spur appears either as a triangular wedge of soft tissue or, when sectioned along its length, as a linear septum that separates adjacent airways or faint curvilinear densities.[45]

After branching off the pulmonary artery below the aortic arch, the right pulmonary artery enters the lung anterior to the right main bronchus; the left pulmonary artery passes above the main

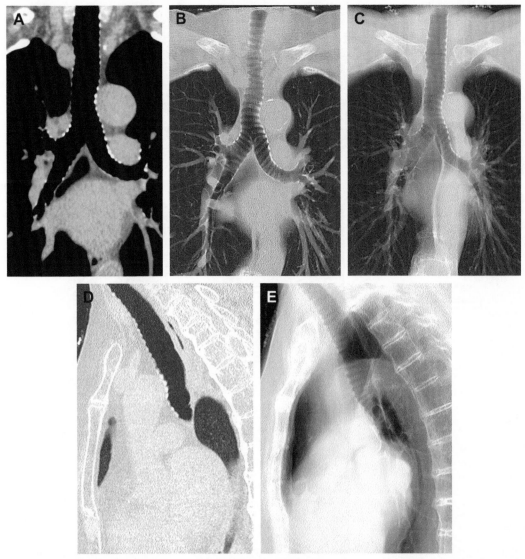

Fig. 8. Single (A), 3-mm (B), and 11-mm (C) slabs average coronal reformats perfectly demonstrate the calcified tracheal rings in a normal older woman. Single (D) and 62-mm (E) slab average sagittal reformats. The lack of cartilage at the level of the posterior wall of the trachea is well seen (arrows). Conversely, the ring cartilages that are partially calcified are obvious at the level of the anterior and lateral part of the trachea (arrows).

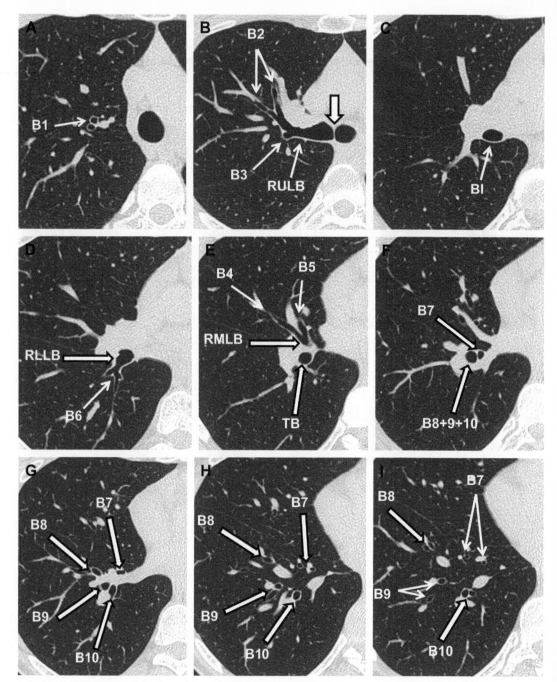

Fig. 9. Normal anatomy of the bronchi on the right side. The first Boyden's classification is used with successive 1-mm slices. (*A*) The arrow shows the division of the apical bronchus of the right upper lobe. Note the oval shape of the normal trachea. (*B*) Right upper lobe bronchus arises from the lateral aspect of the main bronchus, approximately 2 cm distal to the carina (*large arrow*) and courses horizontally for approximately 1 cm from its origin before dividing in segmental branches. Subsegmental bronchi of the anterior bronchus of the right upper lobe are marked by arrows. (*C*) The bronchus intermedius divides after 3 to 4 cm into the middle lobe and lower lobe bronchi. (*D–F*) The middle lobe bronchus arises from the anterolateral wall of the bronchus intermedius and courses anteriorly and laterally for 1 to 2 cm before dividing into lateral (B4) and medial (B5) branches. This origin of the middle lobe is almost at the same level as B6, which is the first branch of the short right lower lobar bronchus (RLLB). The superior segmental bronchus B6 and its subsegmental bronchi arise from the posterior aspect of the RLLB just beyond its origin and course posteriorly. The truncus basalis represents a continuation of the lower lobar bronchus below the origin of B6 and typically appears circular or ovoid. It extends for approximately 1 cm before dividing in four basal segmental bronchi. The first basal bronchi is the medial basilar segmental bronchus (B7) that arises anteromedially from the TB. (*G–I*) Next, there is a successive appearance of the anterior, lateral (B9), and posterior basilar (B10) bronchi and their respective subsegmental bronchi. Note that B7 and its subsegmental bronchus lie typically anterior to the inferior pulmonary vein. (*J*) 3D volume rendering.

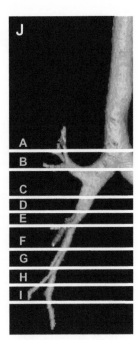

Fig. 9. (*continued*).

stem bronchus and then over the superior lobar bronchus, coming to lie posterior to the bronchus. Within the lung parenchyma, the bronchi and pulmonary artery branches are closely associated and branch in parallel until they reach the acini. Their appearance depends on their orientation. When imaged at an angle to their longitudinal axis, central pulmonary arteries normally appear as rounded or elliptic opacities accompanied by uniformly thin-walled bronchi of similar size and shape. Bronchi and pulmonary arteries appear as cylindrical structures that taper as they branch when imaged along their long axes; they appear rounded if they lie perpendicular to the plane of the CT or elliptical when oriented obliquely. Bronchi and arteries are encased by the peribronchovascular interstitium, which extends from the pulmonary hila into the peripheral lung. The pulmonary veins drain independently from the bronchi with two trunks that enter the left atrium separately.

All conducting airways are muscular tubes lined by a ciliated epithelium. Bronchi with a diameter of approximately 1 mm or more have walls reinforced by cartilage, which take the form of variably shaped islands that diminish in size and number progressively with the decreasing caliber of the bronchi. According to Hayward and Reid,[55] a high density of cartilage was observed for the first four to six generations that effectively provided a circumferential support; the axial bronchi had only scattered plates for another four to six generations. Bronchioles are conducting airways with a wall less than 1 mm in diameter consisting in smooth muscle enclosed in a thin connective tissue space without cartilage. Membranous bronchioles do not contain alveoli, as opposed to respiratory bronchioles, which are lined partly by alveoli. The terminal bronchioles identify the most distal generation of membranous bronchioles, that is, the parent generation to the respiratory bronchioles. Two to three additional generations of respiratory bronchioles are present after the most proximal branch.

The outer diameter of a bronchus is approximately equal to that of the adjacent pulmonary artery. The normal bronchoarterial ratio, defined as the internal diameter (ie, luminal diameter) of the bronchus divided by the diameter of the adjacent pulmonary artery, generally averages 0.65 to 0.70.[56] The presence of a bronchoarterial ratio of more than 1 in normal subjects has been associated with increased age.[56] The measurement has been found to be influenced by altitude, presumably as a result of the combination of hypoxic vasoconstriction and bronchodilatation. In one investigation of 17 normal, nonsmoking individuals living at 1600 m and 16 individuals living at sea level, the mean bronchoarterial ratio was 0.76 at altitude and 0.62 at sea level.[57] The bronchoarterial ratio may also appear to be more than 1 if the scan traverses an undivided bronchus near its branch point and its accompanying artery already has branched.[58]

Anatomically, the walls of large bronchi, outlined by lung on one side and air in the bronchial lumen on the other, appear smooth and of uniform thickness. The normal thickness of an airway wall is related to its diameter, with a normal bronchial wall thickness corresponding to approximately 10% to 30% of the bronchial diameter. Lobar to segmental bronchi (second to fourth generation) have a wall thickness of approximately 1.5 mm and a mean diameter between 5 and 8 mm. Subsegmental (sixth to eighth generation) bronchi have a wall thickness of approximately 0.3 mm and mean diameters between 1.5 and 3 mm. Currently, subsegmental bronchi are routinely identifiable; more distal airways (eleventh to thirteenth generation) have a wall thickness of 0.1 to 0.15 mm and diameters that measure 0.7 to 1 mm.[59] The visibility of normal bronchioles depends on their wall thickness rather than diameter. The smallest airways normally visible using HRCT have a diameter of approximately 2 mm and a wall thickness of 0.2 to 0.3 mm. The value

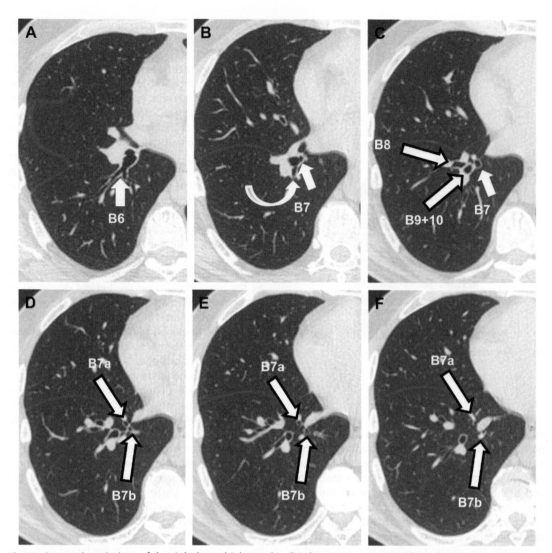

Fig. 10. Anatomic variations of the right bronchial tree. (*A–C*) Subsuperior segmental bronchus B*, accessory superior segmental bronchus or subapical bronchus, is a common variation of the right lower lobe originating below B6 (*A*) at a variable level from the truncus basalis down to the posterior segmental basilar bronchus. In this case, the origin is well seen in (*B*) at the posterior part of the B8 + 9 + 10 trunk (*curved arrow*), B7 lying medially. Successive origin of B8 and B9 + 10 in (*C*). (*D–F*) Most common variation of the subdivision of medial basilar segmental bronchus B7. In this case, the medial ramus B7b courses posterior to the inferior pulmonary vein, unlike the anterior ramus B7a, which remains anterior to the vein.

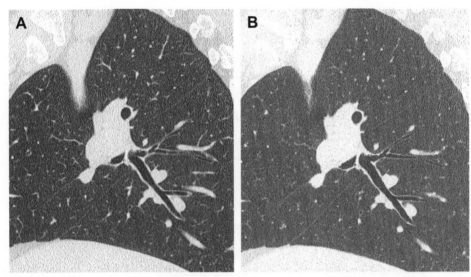

Fig. 11. (*A, B*) Subapical bronchus originates from the posterior basilar segmental bronchus of the right lower lobe. Single reformat (*left*) and thin mIP (*right*) allow visualization of the complete course of B6 and the abnormal bronchi, which have a similar horizontally posterior course.

of the caliber of a bronchiole supplying a secondary lobule, a terminal bronchiole, and a distal respiratory bronchiole is 1 mm, approximately 0.6 mm, and approximately 0.4 mm, respectively, and the thickness of its wall measures approximately 0.15 mm, 0.1 mm, and less than 0.1 mm, respectively.[58] As a result, normal bronchioles are not visible on CT scans. Airways are rarely seen within 1 cm of the pleural surface in most locations, except adjacent to the mediastinum.[57]

CT measurement slightly overestimates wall thickness because it also includes the surrounding peribronchial interstitium. The apparent bronchial wall thickness and diameter of bronchi are markedly influenced by the display parameters. The window and width levels that provide the most accurate measurement of bronchial caliber and wall thickness are −450 to −500 HU and 1000 to 1500 HU, respectively.[29,35,60] When an incorrect parameter is used, the error in estimating the thickness or size of a structure is related to its actual thickness or size, greater fractional overestimates, or underestimates being made for small structures.

In their study, Matsuoka and colleagues[56] found variation of airway caliber and wall area percentage within individual bronchi on cross-sectional CT sections in asymptomatic subjects without cardiopulmonary disease. In 32.7% of the sites observed in contiguous CT sections, the airway lumen did not decrease on the peripheral side, as classically expected. According to the authors, the proportions of epithelium, smooth muscle, interstitial connective tissue,

and cartilage varying at different levels of the bronchus, variation within individual airway lumens, and wall area percentage may be based on variation of bronchial morphology. Quantitative evaluation of the degree of heterogeneous constrictor responses to bronchial challenge should include consideration of normal variation of airway lumen.

Expiratory HRCT may demonstrate lobular areas of air trapping in as many as 60% of normal patients. The prevalence of air trapping increases with age.[61-63] The dependent lung, the lung bases, and the superior segments of the lower lobes are most often concerned. The degree of air trapping that may be identified in normal patients remains controversial, however.

SUMMARY

The new generation of MDCT has revolutionized noninvasive imaging of proximal and distal airways. Exquisite anatomic details of the airway lumen and airway wall on axial CT images benefit in routine practice from postprocessing tools in adequate orientation, ensuring excellent assessment of the morphology and location of any pathologic condition. This technique may be combined with use of low-dose CT. The next challenge for CT is the functional assessment with accurate quantification of caliber and thickness of the whole bronchial tree integrated in the more complex evaluation of the lung parenchyma, including hypoattenuated areas.

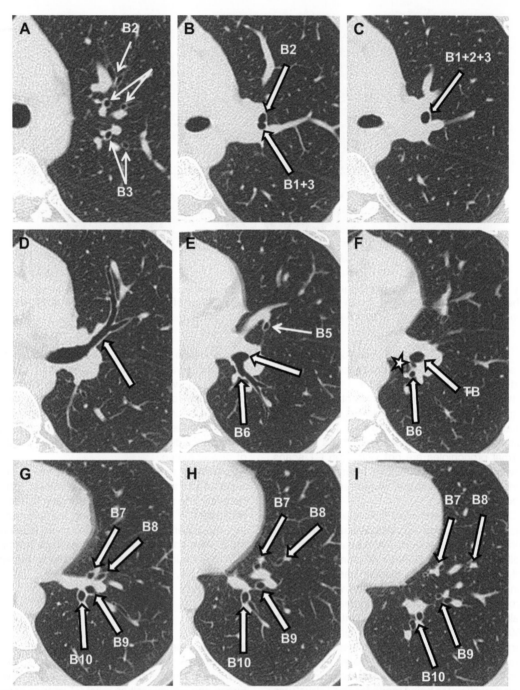

Fig. 12. Normal anatomy of the bronchi on the left side. The first Boyden's classification is used with successive 1-mm slices. (A–C) The left upper lobe bronchus bifurcates in most cases in an upper culminal bronchus (CB), which almost immediately divides into an apicoposterior (B1 + 3) and anterior (B2) segmental bronchus and in a lower division, the lingular bronchus. (A) Subsegmental divisions of B1, B2, B3 are shown (arrows). (D–F) The lingular bronchus (arrow in D) arises from the lower part of the left upper lobar bronchus (LULB), extends anteriorly and inferiorly for 2 to 3 cm, and then bifurcates into the superior (B4) and inferior divisions (B5). The course of B4 tends to be more lateral and horizontal than B5. Left lower lobar bronchus (LLLB) and B6 are similar to those on the right side. (F) Note that the rounded lucency corresponds to the medial subsegmental branch of B6 and that the lucency at the posterior part of the TB (star) corresponds to a subapical branch of the LLLB, more rarely seen on the left side than on the right side. (G–I) The truncus basalis is longer than on the right side and divides into three basal segmental bronchi, including anteromedial (B7 + 8), lateral (B9), and posterior (B10). (J) 3D volume rendering.

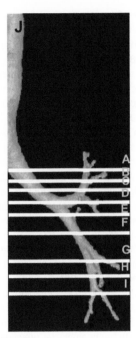

Fig. 12. (*continued*).

REFERENCES

1. Beigelman-Aubry C, Hill C, Guibal A, et al. Multi-detector row CT and postprocessing techniques in the assessment of diffuse lung disease. Radiographics 2005;25:1639–52.

2. Grenier PA, Beigelman-Aubry C, Fetita C, et al. New frontiers in CT imaging of airway disease. Eur Radiol 2002;12:1022–44.

3. LoCicero J 3rd, Costello P, Campos CT, et al. Spiral CT with multiplanar and three-dimensional reconstructions accurately predicts tracheobronchial pathology. Ann Thorac Surg 1996;62:811–7.

4. Remy-Jardin M, Remy J, Deschildre F, et al. Obstructive lesions of the central airways: evaluation by using spiral CT with multiplanar and three-dimensional reformations. Eur Radiol 1996;6:807–16.

5. Beigelman-Aubry C. Post-processing and display in multislice CT of the chest. JBR-BTR 2007;90:85–8.

6. Arakawa H, Sasaka K, Lu WM, et al. Comparison of axial high-resolution CT and thin-section multiplanar reformation (MPR) for diagnosis of diseases of the pulmonary parenchyma: preliminary study in 49 patients. J Thorac Imaging 2004;19:24–31.

7. Remy J, Remy-Jardin M, Artaud D, et al. Multiplanar and three-dimensional reconstruction techniques in CT: impact on chest diseases. Eur Radiol 1998;8:335–51.

8. Salvolini L, Bichi Secchi E, Costarelli L, et al. Clinical applications of 2D and 3D CT imaging of the airways: a review. Eur J Radiol 2000;34:9–25.

9. Fraser RS, Muller NL, Colman N, et al. The normal lung: computed tomography. In: Fraser RS, Muller NL, Colman N, et al, editors. Diagnosis of diseases of the chest. 4th edition. Philadelphia: WB Saunders; 1999. p. 281–95.

10. Bhalla M, Naidich DP, McGuinness G, et al. Diffuse lung disease: assessment with helical CT. Preliminary observations of the role of maximum and minimum intensity projection images. Radiology 1996;200:341–7.

11. Remy-Jardin M, Remy J, Artaud D, et al. Diffuse infiltrative lung disease: clinical value of sliding-thin-slab maximum intensity projection CT scans in the detection of mild micronodular patterns. Radiology 1996;200:333–9.

12. Gruden JF, Ouanounou S, Tigges S, et al. Incremental benefit of maximum-intensity-projection images on observer detection of small pulmonary nodules revealed by multidetector CT. AJR Am J Roentgenol 2002;179:149–57.

13. Boiselle PM, Lynch DA. Anatomical airway imaging methods. In: Boiselle PM, Lynch DA, editors. CT of the airways. Totowa (NJ): Humana Press; 2008. p. 75–94.

14. Remy-Jardin M, Remy J, Artaud D, et al. Volume rendering of the tracheobronchial tree: clinical evaluation of bronchographic images. Radiology 1998; 208:761–70.

15. Kauczor HU, Hofmann D, Kreitner KF, et al. Normal and abnormal pulmonary ventilation: visualization at hyperpolarized He-3 MR imaging. Radiology 1996;201:564–8.

16. Fetita C, Preteux F, Beigelman-Aubry C, et al. 3D bronchoview: a new software package for investigating airway diseases. [abstract]. Eur Radiol 2002;12:394.

17. Hopper KD, Iyriboz TA, Mahraj RP, et al. CT bronchoscopy: optimization of imaging parameters. Radiology 1998;209:872–7.

18. Boiselle PM, Reynolds KF, Ernst A. Multiplanar and three-dimensional imaging of the central airways with multidetector CT. AJR Am J Roentgenol 2002; 179:301–8.

19. Summers RM, Selbie WS, Malley JD, et al. Polypoid lesions of airways: early experience with computer-assisted detection by using virtual bronchoscopy and surface curvature. Radiology 1998; 208:331–7.

20. Newmark GM, Conces DJ Jr, Kopecky KK. Spiral CT evaluation of the trachea and bronchi. J Comput Assist Tomogr 1994;18:552–4.

21. Ferretti GR, Bricault I, Coulomb M. Virtual tools for imaging of the thorax. Eur Respir J 2001;18: 381–92.

22. Newman KB, Lynch DA, Newman LS, et al. Quantitative computed tomography detects air trapping due to asthma. Chest 1994;106:105–9.

23. Zhang J, Hasegawa I, Hatabu H, et al. Frequency and severity of air trapping at dynamic expiratory CT in patients with tracheobronchomalacia. AJR Am J Roentgenol 2004;182:81–5.

24. Wittram C, Batt J, Rappaport DC, et al. Inspiratory and expiratory helical CT of normal adults: comparison of thin section scans and minimum intensity projection images. J Thorac Imaging 2002;17:47–52.

25. Nishino M, Hatabu H. Volumetric expiratory HRCT imaging with MSCT. J Thorac Imaging 2005;20: 176–85.

26. Fetita CI, Preteux F, Beigelman-Aubry C, et al. Pulmonary airways: 3-D reconstruction from multi-slice CT and clinical investigation. IEEE Trans Med Imaging 2004;23:1353–64.

27. Amirav I, Kramer SS, Grunstein MM, et al. Assessment of methacholine-induced airway constriction by ultrafast high-resolution computed tomography. J Appl Phys 1993;75:2239–50.

28. King GG, Muller NL, Whittall KP, et al. An analysis algorithm for measuring airway lumen and wall areas from high-resolution computed tomographic data. Am J Respir Crit Care Med 2000;161:574–80.

29. McNamara AE, Muller NL, Okazawa M, et al. Airway narrowing in excised canine lungs measured by high-resolution computed tomography. J Appl Phys 1992;73:307–16.

30. Perot V, Desberat P, Berger P, et al. Nouvel algorithme d'extraction des paramètres géométriques des bronches en TDMHR. [abstract]. J Radiol 2001;82:1213 [in French].

31. Prêteux F, Fetita CI, Capderou A, et al. Modeling, segmentation, and caliber estimation of bronchi in high resolution computerized tomography. J Electron Imaging 1999;8:36–45.

32. Wood SA, Zerhouni EA, Hoford JD, et al. Measurement of three-dimensional lung tree structures by using computed tomography. J Appl Phys 1995; 79:1687–97.

33. Okazawa M, Muller N, McNamara AE, et al. Human airway narrowing measured using high resolution computed tomography. Am J Respir Crit Care Med 1996;154:1557–62.

34. Seneterre E, Paganin F, Bruel JM, et al. Measurement of the internal size of bronchi using high resolution computed tomography (HRCT). Eur Respir J 1994;7:596–600.

35. Webb WR, Gamsu G, Wall SD, et al. CT of a bronchial phantom: factors affecting appearance and size measurements. Invest Radiol 1984;19:394–8.

36. Beigelman-Aubry C, Capderou A, Grenier PA, et al. Mild intermittent asthma: CT assessment of bronchial cross-sectional area and lung attenuation at controlled lung volume. Radiology 2002;223:181–7.

37. Brown R, Mitzner W, Bulut Y, et al. Effect of lung inflation in vivo on airways with smooth-muscle tone or edema. J Appl Phys 1997;82(2):491–9.

38. Brown RH, Georgakopoulos J, Mitzner W. Individual canine airways responsiveness to aerosol histamine and methacholine in vivo. Am J Respir Crit Care Med 1998;157:491–7.

39. King GG, Muller NL, Pare PD. Evaluation of airways in obstructive pulmonary disease using high-resolution computed tomography. Am J Respir Crit Care Med 1999;159:992–1004.

40. Nakano Y, Muro S, Sakai H, et al. Computed tomographic measurements of airway dimensions and emphysema in smokers: correlation with lung function. Am J Respir Crit Care Med 2000;162:1102–8.

41. Niimi A, Matsumoto H, Amitani R, et al. Airway wall thickness in asthma assessed by computed tomography: relation to clinical indices. Am J Respir Crit Care Med 2000;162:1518–23.

42. Gamsu G, Webb WR. Computed tomography of the trachea: normal and abnormal. AJR Am J Roentgenol 1982;139:321–6.

43. Holbert JM, Strollo DC. Imaging of the normal trachea. J Thorac Imaging 1995;10:171–9.

44. Boiselle PM, Ernst A. Tracheal morphology in patients with tracheomalacia: prevalence of inspiratory lunate and expiratory "frown" shapes. J Thorac Imaging 2006;21:190–6.

45. Naidich D, Webb WR, Grenier PA, et al. Introduction to imaging methodology and airway anatomy. In: Naidich D, Webb WR, Grenier PA, Harkin TJ, Gefter WB, editors. Imaging of the airways: functional and radiologic correlations. Philadelphia: Lippincott Williams & Wilkins; 2005. p. 1–28.

46. Boiselle PM, Lynch DA. Radiologic anatomy of the airways. In: Boiselle PM, Lynch DA, editors. CT of the airways. Totowa (NJ): Humana Press; 2008. p. 25–48.

47. Vock P, Spiegel T, Fram EK, et al. CT assessment of the adult intrathoracic cross section of the trachea. J Comput Assist Tomogr 1984;8:1076–82.

48. Breatnach E, Abbott GC, Fraser RG. Dimensions of the normal human trachea. AJR Am J Roentgenol 1984;142:903–6.

49. Woodring JH, Howard RS 2nd, Rehm SR. Congenital tracheobronchomegaly (Mounier-Kuhn syndrome): a report of 10 cases and review of the literature. J Thorac Imaging 1991;6:1–10.

50. Webb EM, Elicker BM, Webb WR. Using CT to diagnose nonneoplastic tracheal abnormalities: appearance of the tracheal wall. AJR Am J Roentgenol 2000;174:1315–21.

51. Olivier P, Hayon-Sonsino D, Convard JP, et al. Measurement of left mainstem bronchus using multiplane CT reconstructions and relationship between patient characteristics or tracheal diameters and left bronchial diameters. Chest 2006;130: 101–7.

52. Thurlbeck WM, Churg AM. Pathology of the lung. New York: Thieme Medical Publishers; 1995.

53. Boyden EA. The nomenclature of the bronchopulmonary segments and their blood supply. Dis Chest
1961;39:1–6.

54. Jackson CI, Huber JF. Correlated applied anatomy
of the bronchial tree and lungs with a system of
nomenclature. Dis Chest 1943;9:319–26.

55. Hayward J, Reid ML. The cartilage of the intra-
pulmonary bronchi in normal lungs, in bronchiectasis, and in massive collapse. Thorax 1952;7:
98–110.

56. Matsuoka S, Kurihara Y, Nakajima Y, et al. Serial
change in airway lumen and wall thickness at thin-
section CT in asymptomatic subjects. Radiology
2005;234:595–603.

57. Kim JS, Muller NL, Park CS, et al. Bronchoarterial
ratio on thin section CT: comparison between high
altitude and sea level. J Comput Assist Tomogr
1997;21:306–11.

58. Webb WR, Müller NL, Naidich DP. Normal lung
anatomy. In: High-resolution CT of the lung. 3rd
edition. Philadelphia: Lippincott Wiliams & Wilkins;
2009. p. 42–64.

59. Weibel ER. High resolution computed tomography of
the pulmonary parenchyma: anatomical background. Presented at the Fleiszchner Society
Symposium on Chest Disease. Scottsdale, AZ, April
21, 1990.

60. Bankier AA, Fleischmann D, Mallek R, et al. Bronchial wall thickness: appropriate window settings
for thin-section CT and radiologic-anatomic correlation. Radiology 1996;199:831–6.

61. Mastora I, Remy-Jardin M, Sobaszek A, et al. Thin-
section CT finding in 250 volunteers: assessment
of the relationship of CT findings with smoking
history and pulmonary function test results. Radiology 2001;218:695–702.

62. Tanaka N, Matsumoto T, Miura G, et al. Air trapping
at CT: high prevalence in asymptomatic subjects
with normal pulmonary function. Radiology 2003;
227:776–85.

63. Lee KW, Chung SY, Yang I, et al. Correlation of aging
and smoking with air trapping at thin-section CT of
the lung in asymptomatic subjects. Radiology
2000;214:831–6.

Congenital Abnormalities of Intrathoracic Airways

Amandine Desir, MD, Benoît Ghaye, MD*

KEYWORDS
• Computed tomography (CT) helical • Bronchi abnormalities
• Bronchi CT • Trachea abnormalities • Lung anatomy

In the past, congenital tracheobronchial variants or anomalies were demonstrated in 1% to 12% of patients at bronchography or bronchoscopy.[1–3] Anomalies of the tracheobronchial tree are diagnosed with increasing frequency as a result of refinement in contemporary imaging and classification. Multidetector CT (MDCT) has broadened the potential of imaging of lung anatomy, offering different modalities of reformatting which improve the understanding of complex tracheobronchial anomalies, even in the pediatric population.[4–12] Most congenital tracheobronchial anomalies are rare and almost always nonsymptomatic. Nevertheless, such anomalies are important to know because some may be confused with or even responsible for respiratory disease. They may also be associated with cardiovascular and/or other organ malformations;[13] furthermore, radiologists should be familiar with anatomic variants and anomalies to guide adequately clinicians or surgeons when bronchoscopy or surgical planning is needed.

EMBRYOLOGY

Normal tracheobronchial development is initiated at 24 to 26 days as a median bulge of the ventral wall of the pharynx which develops at the caudal end of the laryngotracheal groove. At 26 to 28 days, it gives rise to right and left lung buds. As the lung buds elongate, the trachea is separated from the esophagus by lateral ingrowth of the mesoderm forming the tracheoesophageal septum. The endodermal lining of the laryngotracheal tube gives rise to the epithelium of the tracheobronchial tree, whereas cartilage, connective tissue, and muscle develop from the surrounding splanchnic mesenchyme. By 28 to 30 days, the lung buds have elongated into primary bronchi. The five lobar bronchi have appeared by 30 to 32 days, and all segmental bronchi are formed by 36 days. Over the same period, the vascular supply to this tissue shifts from branches of the splenic plexus to define the pulmonary artery (PA) as fusion of the lung bud plexus with the sixth branchial arches occurs.[13]

Three major hypotheses have been formulated to explain the pathogenesis of anomalous tracheobronchial development.[14,15] The reduction theory postulates that the final anatomy is the result of shrinkage and finally suppression of portions of a primitive pattern encompassing all the components of the extant mammalian bronchial distribution.[16] The migration theory considers that bronchial outgrowths have the potential of migrating from their initial locus to new points of origin of a bronchus or the trachea. The selection theory advocates local disturbances in the development during budding of the bronchial buds under the influence of bronchial mesenchyma.[17] It is likely that defects involving supernumerary tracheal bronchi occur early in the development around 29 to 30 days as the lobar bronchi start to differentiate. On the other hand, displaced bronchi would more likely occur after 32 days as the bronchi elongate and branch further.[14] Various hypotheses have been proposed to explain anomalous communications between the esophagus and tracheobronchial tree.[9,18]

Department of Medical Imaging, University Hospital of Liège, B35 Sart Tilman, B-4000 Liège, Belgium
* Corresponding author.
E-mail address: bghaye@chu.ulg.ac.be (B. Ghaye).

Radiol Clin N Am 47 (2009) 203–225
doi:10.1016/j.rcl.2008.11.009
0033-8389/08/$ – see front matter © 2009 Elsevier Inc. All rights reserved.

DEVELOPMENTAL INTERRUPTION

Congenital underdevelopment of the tracheobronchial tree and the lungs, known as the agenesis-hypoplasia complex, has been classified into three groups according to the embryologic stage of developmental interruption: (1) agenesis (absence of bronchus, vessel, and lung parenchyma), (2) aplasia (absence of lung parenchyma with blind rudimentary bronchus present), and (3) hypoplasia (decrease of the number and size of bronchi, vessels, and parenchymal structures).[19] Diagnosis is easily established when related to a whole lung or lobe but can be more difficult when related to segmental bronchi (Fig. 1).

Tracheal agenesis/aplasia is an exceptional malformation due to failure of development of the lung bud resulting in complete absence of the trachea and lungs, not compatible with life.

Pulmonary agenesis and aplasia can affect both lungs with similar frequency and may remain asymptomatic, leading to incidental discovery in adults.[19–23] When symptoms are present, respiratory distress or recurrent infections are more frequently reported in agenesis or aplasia of the right lung, probably due to greater mechanical compression and distortion of bronchial and vascular structures secondary to an ipsilateral rotation of the mediastinum.[22,23] Recurrent infections may be even more frequent in patients with aplasia of one lung, with the blind bronchus potentially acting as a reservoir.[20,24] Vestigial lung parenchyma can be found at the end of the aplastic bronchus.[25] Associated malformations are reported in half of patients.[19,22,23] Lung hypoplasia is generally secondary (ie, to a neighboring space-occupying lesion or malformation that stunts lung growth).[22,23]

Lobar and segmental agenesis or aplasia is more frequently found in the right upper lobe (RUL). When isolated, it is usually asymptomatic (see Fig. 1). Lobar hypoplasia may be seen in various

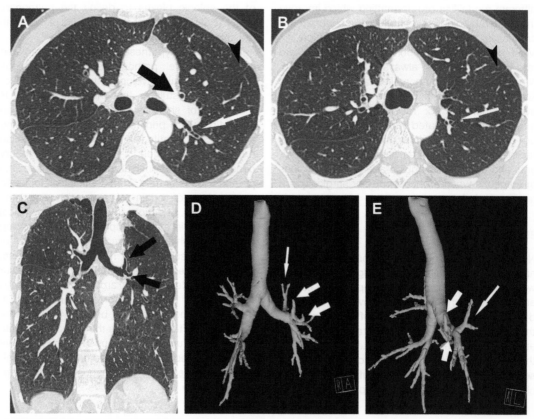

Fig. 1. Aplasia of segmental bronchi of the left upper lobe. (A–E) Axial CT slices, coronal MPR, and three-dimensional volume-rendering reformatting show blind anterior and apicoposterior segmental bronchi (*arrows*) of the left upper lobe. The left lung is smaller than the right one, and the left major fissure (*arrowheads*) is displaced anteriorly due to moderate hypoplasia of the left upper lobe. The apex of the left lung is ventilated by the superior segmental bronchus of the left lower lobe (*long arrow*). MPR, multiplanar reformatting.

conditions, including bronchial atresia, bridging bronchus (BB), esophageal bronchus, and congenital bronchial stenosis, or in patients with an ipsilateral vascular malformation such as in the hypogenetic lung syndrome or veno-lobar syndrome.[11,19,22–24] Congenital bronchiectasis is a rare disease manifesting as tubular dilatation of all bronchi in a lobe or a lung extending up to the pleural surface and associated with focal lung hypoplasia. It has been hypothesized to be secondary to incomplete branching of the developing bronchial tree.[26]

COMMUNICATING BRONCHOPULMONARY FOREGUT MALFORMATIONS—ESOPHAGEAL BRONCHUS

Communicating bronchopulmonary foregut malformations (CBPFMs) are uncommon anomalies characterized by a patent congenital communication between a portion of respiratory tract on one side and the esophagus or stomach on the other side.[27–32] Concomitant congenital tracheobronchial stenoses have been reported.[33,34] CBPFMs can also occur in combination with other congenital anomalies involving the pulmonary and systemic vascular systems, diaphragm, upper gastrointestinal tract, and rib and vertebrae.[28,30,35]

A classification of CBPFMs into four groups has been proposed by Srikanth based on anatomic features and how the lung bud joins the esophagus.[31] The first group comprises an esophageal atresia, with the distal gastroesophageal tract originating from the trachea, a condition generally readily diagnosed in neonates.[5,30,33] One lung, lobe, or segment then arises from the distal esophagus. The three other groups encompass communicating malformations without esophageal atresia and with variable blood supply. Malformations in the second and the third groups are the most frequent, being reported in 33% and 46% of patients presenting with CBPFMS, respectively.[31] In the second group, one whole lung originates from the esophagus and is generally termed an *esophageal lung* or *accessory lung*.[27,35,36] Ninety-five percent of esophageal lungs are right sided.[31] The ipsilateral main bronchus is absent, resulting in complete absence of ventilatory function of the involved lung that is hypoplastic and atelectated.[34] Malformations in the third group are characterized by a single lobe or segment arising from the esophagus or the stomach.[30] The bronchus originating from the gastrointestinal tract is classically called an "esophageal bronchus" (**Fig. 2**).[32,36] Exceptional bilateral esophageal bronchi have been reported.[27,37] In the fourth group, there is a simple communication between a portion of

the bronchial system and the esophagus and a systemic vascular supply.[31] Another classification of CBPFMs based on the morphology of the fistulous tract (neck, diverticulum, cyst) and the blood supply has also been proposed.[38] The most common communications are between the mid- or distal third of the esophagus and the right lower lobe (RLL) (43%), left lower lobe (LLL) (22%), or right main bronchus (RMB) (10%).[39]

The clinical course of CBPFMs is generally insidious, including cough, recurrent pneumonia, and hemoptysis owing to chronic bronchopulmonary infection.[27,32,39,40] Episodes of choking when swallowing liquids or the presence of food particles in sputum are suggestive and reported in 65% of patients.[32,38–40] Nevertheless, the diagnosis is not made before adulthood in approximately 75% of cases.[39,40] Various hypotheses concerning the late diagnosis have been proposed, including a late onset or intermittence of symptoms or mild complaints leading to delayed investigation only after the development of complications. The late appearance of symptoms may result from the presence of a membrane or valve within the fistulous tract that subsequently ruptures or becomes incompetent,[29,39] the oblique upwards course of the fistula,[40] or the closure or contraction of the fistula during swallowing.[29,40] Diagnosis is usually made by barium esophagography together with bronchial and esophageal endoscopy.[7,30,36,40,41] In addition to the fistulous tract, CT may demonstrate bronchiectasis, rudimentary lung tissue, and zones of consolidation and fibrosis in the area "ventilated" by the anomalous bronchus and may also map vascular supply and drainage.[7,32,42] Furthermore, three-dimensional CT esophagography may help to evidence the communication and display complex anatomic features.[5,41,43] The differential diagnosis includes pulmonary sequestration, congenital cystic adenomatoid malformation (CCAM), and iatrogenic, inflammatory, or neoplastic fistulas.[32] Treatment consists of either resection of the esophageal lung, or lobe, or anastomosis of the esophageal lung with the normal tracheobronchial tree when there is no severe broncho-parenchymal lesion and the vascular supply is normal.[36]

CONGENITAL OBSTRUCTION OR COMPRESSION
Tracheal Atresia

Tracheal atresia is an exceptional anomaly in which a segment of the trachea, generally proximal, is missing.[9] The anomaly is lethal except when associated with a tracheo-esophageal fistula, allowing esophageal intubation and subsequent surgical reconstruction.[9,44] Three types of

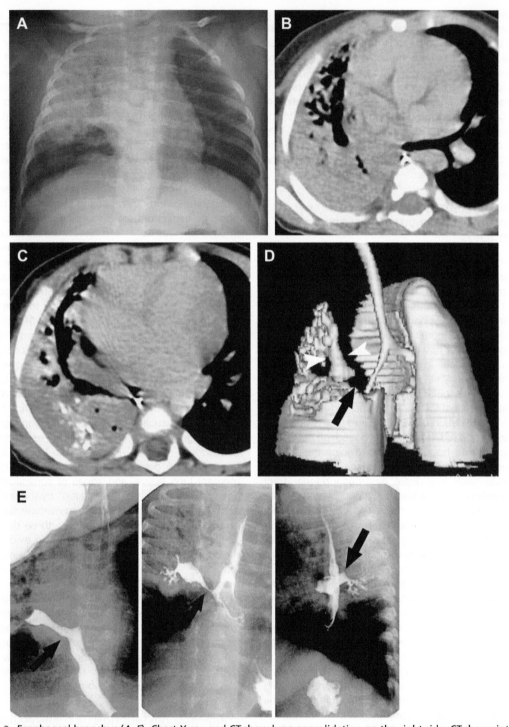

Fig. 2. Esophageal bronchus (*A–E*). Chest X-ray and CT show lung consolidation on the right side. CT shows intra-pulmonary contrast after esophagram. Esophagram shows aberrant bronchus arising from the esophagus (*arrows*). Three-dimensional volume rendered image shows esophageal bronchus (*arrow*) and esophageal lobe (*arrowheads*). (*Courtesy of* Woo Sun Kim, MD, Seoul, Korea).

tracheal atresia have been described depending on the tracheobronchial segment that communicates with esophagus, with the carina being the most frequent (60%) site of communication.[9,20,45] Prenatal diagnosis of such malformations has virtually never been reported, and CT is helpful in demonstrating their complex anatomy before possible surgery.[9]

Bronchial Atresia

First described by Ramsay and Byron in 1953, bronchial atresia results from a focal and juxtahilar interruption of a segmental (more rarely lobar or subsegmental) bronchus, associated with normal development of the distal airways.[46–51] The left upper lobe (LUL) is most commonly involved (two thirds of patients), particularly the apicoposterior segmental bronchus. The other lobes are more uncommonly affected, with the RUL, LLL, middle lobe (ML), and RLL in descending order.[6,47,48,52–54] Involvement of multiple lung segments has rarely been reported.[48,55]

The origin of bronchial atresia is not known, but most authors suggest that it is congenital. Two main hypotheses have been proposed. The first sug-gests an ischemic insult to a focal portion of the bronchial wall, whereas the second suggests a disconnection from the bronchial bud of a distal group of dividing bronchial cells. The separated cell mass then continues to divide normally, resulting in the normal branching pattern distal to atresia.[47,48,54,56]

The bronchi distal to the site of atresia become filled with mucus not removable by ciliary action and are progressively dilated, forming a bronchocele (Fig. 3). Generally, no connection is found between the bronchocele and the proximal airway, but a fibrous strand may sometimes be present.[47,48,57] The alveoli distal to the atresia are ventilated through collateral pathways and show features of air trapping, resulting in focal hyperinflation.[6,47,50,53,57]

Radiographic features may be highly suggestive of the diagnosis, consisting of central opacities that may show an air-fluid level surrounded by a systematized hyperlucency due to oligemia and air trapping.[47,48,50] Bronchoceles and hyperinflation are seen together only in 57% to 83% of cases.[47,48,50,52,54] CT is the most sensitive method for showing the tubular, ramified, or nodular bronchocele and the distal areas of oligemia and air trapping, which can be more clearly depicted at expiratory CT.[22,25,49,50,54] In lobar atresia with complete fissure, hyperinflation can be missing due to the absence of collateral pathways of ventilation and be replaced by atelectasis or a cystic

lobe.[58] On the other hand, when fissures are incomplete, collateral ventilation may be responsible for huge dilatation of lung parenchyma distal to the lobar atresia and severe compression of normal lung tissue.[51] Systemic arterial supply to the anomalous area simulating a pulmonary sequestration has been reported.[59] MR imaging can demonstrate the bronchocele, showing high signal intensities on T1- and T2-weighted images in 86% of patients.[50] Prenatal identification by sonography and MR imaging has been an important contributor to the marked increase of bronchial atresia in the last decade.[51]

Most patients with bronchial atresia are asymptomatic, but dyspnea, pain, recurrent pneumonia (up to 20% of patients) or pneumothorax, hemoptysis, and asthma have been reported.[47–49,60] The diagnosis is incidental in approximately 50% to 60% of cases, mostly in men during the second or third decade.[6,47,48,50,53] When diagnosed in young children, the clinical presentation may be more severe, including cases of respiratory distress.[47,51,55] Treatment is usually conservative, with surgery only indicated when major clinical symptoms are present.[48–51,55,60]

The differential diagnosis of the bronchocele-hyperlucency syndrome includes an acquired bronchocele, such as in association with bronchiectasis or allergic bronchopulmonary aspergillosis, or may be secondary to bronchial obstruction by tumor, foreign body, external compression, or broncholithiasis. Hyperlucency can also suggest congenital lobar emphysema, CCAM, bronchogenic cyst, pulmonary sequestration, or acquired diseases as the MacLeod syndrome.[25,57] Some of those malformations may also be associated with bronchial atresia.[48,51,54,61] Fiberoptic bronchoscopy is usually normal in bronchial atresia, although sometimes a blind bronchus may be identified.[49,55]

Tracheal and Bronchial Stenosis

Congenital tracheobronchial stenosis corresponds to a more than 50% reduction of the luminal diameter.[44] Primary tracheobronchial stenosis can result from various anomalies of the tracheobronchial wall or from an intraluminal diaphragm.[10,62] Disproportionate development of the cartilage relative to the membranous part may result in absent, hypoplastic, near-complete, or complete cartilaginous rings, or less often in other complex patterns of cartilaginous malformations responsible for stenosis or malacia.[44,62,63] Dynamic MDCT performed during inspiration and expiration is helpful to differentiate stenosis and malacia.[12] Primary tracheal stenoses are divided into three types. The first type (30%) corresponds to a diffuse stenosis of the trachea,

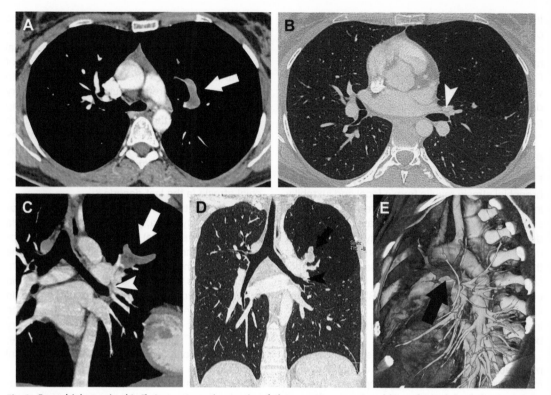

Fig. 3. Bronchial atresia. (*A–E*) Asymptomatic atresia of the anterior segmental bronchus of the left upper lobe (*arrowheads*). Note the large central bronchocele (*arrows*) and localized air-trapping distal to occlusion. Fiberoptic bronchoscopy was normal. The patient was treated conservatively.

the second type (20%) to a "funnel-like" or progressive stenosis of various lengths and locations, and the third type (50%) to a segmental stenosis.[20,53] Long-segment tracheobronchial stenosis due to complete cartilaginous rings is commonly found in patients with a sling of left PA (SLPA) (ring-sling complex) and represents a factor of worse prognosis even after surgery.[64–66]

Secondary tracheobronchial stenoses are related to tracheal compression of various causes, particularly vascular malformations including vascular rings, a dilated or displaced innominate artery, SLPA, cardiac disease, and mediastinal masses.[10,44,62,67] Tracheobronchial stenoses are also reported in patients with congenital lobar emphysema and congenital pulmonary venolobar syndrome.[23,24]

Tracheal Dilatation

Congenital tracheobronchomegaly, also called Mounier-Kuhn syndrome or mega trachea, is characterized by an intrinsic weakness or flaccidity of the wall of the trachea and central bronchi leading to tracheobronchial dilatation at inspiration and collapse at expiration and to formation of diverticula.[68]

ECTOPIC OR SUPERNUMERARY LUNG BUDS

Noncommunicating bronchopulmonary foregut malformations, including among others bronchogenic cysts, result from abnormal budding of the developing tracheobronchial tree. Pulmonary sequestration, CCAM, and congenital lobar emphysema are diseases of lung tissue.[23,25,26] Those anomalies are beyond the scope of this article and are not discussed further herein.

Tracheobronchial Diverticulum

Congenital diverticula are rare and considered to be remnants of an aborted division of the primary lung bud.[69] They are more frequently reported at the level of the trachea than at the bronchi. A tracheal bronchus (TB) and accessory cardiac bronchus (ACB) may present as diverticulum.[3,69,70] Tracheal congenital diverticula usually arise on the right side, 4 or 5 cm below the true vocal cords or a few centimeters above the carina. They are directed obliquely downward and filled with air or mucus (**Fig. 4**).[69,71,72] Histologically, congenital tracheal diverticula are composed of normal tracheal elements such as muscle or cartilage.[69] Associated congenital tracheo-esophageal

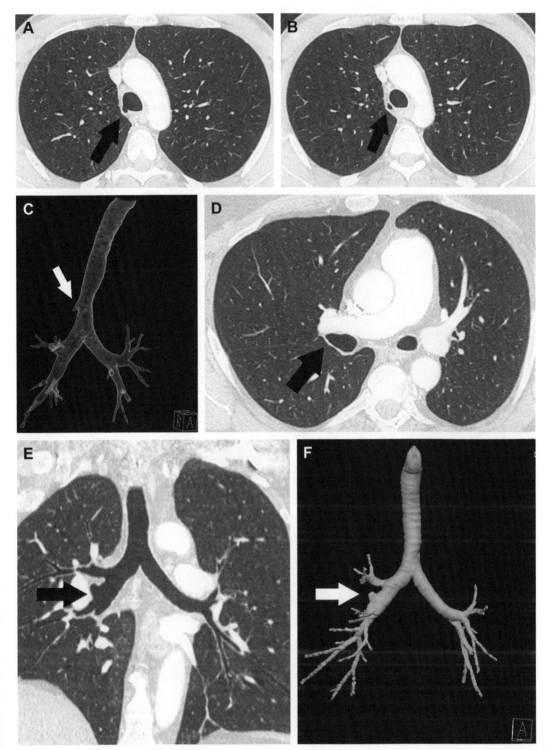

Fig. 4. Congenital diverticulum. (*A–C*) Blind diverticulum filled with air arising from the posterolateral aspect of the right tracheal wall and directing obliquely downwards (*arrows*). According to its location, it may correspond to a blind tracheal bronchus. (*D–F*) Blind diverticulum arising from inferior part of the lateral wall of the intermediate bronchus (*arrows*).

fistula, tracheal stenosis, and CCAM have been reported.[69,71,73]

The main differential diagnoses of congenital tracheobronchial diverticula are acquired diverticula of various forms, including a tracheocele and air-filled hypertrophic adenoid recess (Fig. 5). Paratracheobronchial structures containing air should also be differentiated from laryngocele,

pharyngocele, Zenker's diverticulum, lymphoepithelial cyst, bronchogenic cyst, and apical lung hernia or bulla.[74,75]

Acquired diverticula correspond to simple evaginations of the mucosa through a weak point located laterally between the cartilaginous rings or posterolaterally through the trachealis or bronchialis muscle. They are devoid of smooth

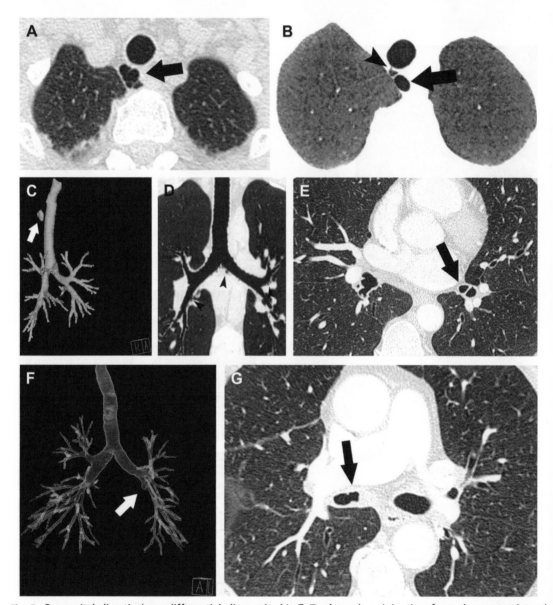

Fig. 5. Congenital diverticulum, differential diagnosis. (*A–C*) Tracheocele originating from the posterolateral aspect of the trachea at the level of T2. Note the small communication between the diverticulum and the trachea on axial minimum intensity projection reformat (*arrowhead*). (*D*) Multiple adenoid recesses filled with air originating from main, lobar, or segmental bronchi (*arrowheads*). (*E–F*) Probably acquired diverticulum originating from the left lower lobe bronchus (*arrow*). It mimics a left-sided blind accessory cardiac bronchus, but no cartilage was demonstrated inside its wall at fiberoptic bronchoscopy. (*G*) Acquired bronchial fistula due to tuberculosis lymphadenopathy. Note small irregularities in the wall contour of the fistulous structure.

muscle or cartilage.[71,76] When developing post-erolaterally, they are almost invariably located on the right side at the level of the thoracic inlet and are termed *tracheoceles*.[74,76,77] Tracheoceles are generally single and larger than other acquired diverticula.[75] When developing laterally, acquired diverticula can occur on both sides, mainly at the bronchial level. These 1- to 3-mm outpouchings may be single or multiple, as frequently seen in association with chronic

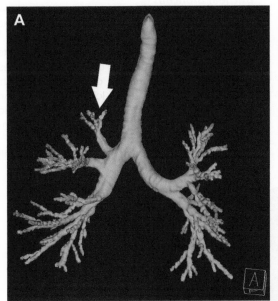

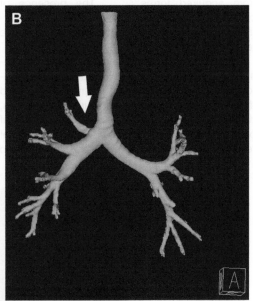

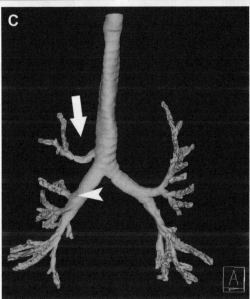

Fig. 6. Right tracheal bronchi. Volume-rendering CT bronchography showing the three typical locations of tracheal bronchi (*arrows*). All tracheal bronchi are displaced and pre-eparterial type. (*A*) Tracheal bronchus originating from the right main bronchus, also called double-right superior lobe bronchus in this location. The tracheal bronchus corresponds to a displaced superior segmental bronchus (B1) of the right upper lobe. (*B*) Tracheal bronchus originating from the carina, also corresponding to a displaced B1. (*C*) Tracheal bronchus originating from the trachea, also called "pig bronchus" in this location, which is the most caricatural but less common presentation of a tracheal bronchus. The tracheal bronchus gives B1 (superior segmental bronchus) and B2 (anterior segmental bronchus). B3 (posterior segmental bronchus) is displaced downward on the intermediate bronchus (*arrowhead*).

obstructive pulmonary disease, or even as a diverticulosis in Mounier-Kuhn disease.[77,78] Other acquired diverticula may be secondary to traction phenomena, usually in relation with adenopathy or pulmonary fibrosis. Considering the shape of the mouth, number, or size of diverticula is not sufficient to differentiate congenital from acquired forms.[72,75,79] The presence of cartilage may suggest a congenital origin. Nevertheless, it remains difficult to demonstrate these features with CT.[72]

Congenital diverticula are generally asymptomatic but sometimes present with nonspecific symptoms related to any form of inflamed or infected diverticula, such as chronic cough, hemoptysis, dyspnea, and stridor, and as repetitive episodes of bronchopulmonary infections.[69,72,75] A case of recurrent laryngeal nerve paralysis secondary to compression from a tracheal congenital diverticulum has been reported.[72] Ineffective ventilation or pneumomediastinum secondary to accidental perforation of a diverticulum after tracheal intubation has also been described.[69,72,75]

Tracheal Bronchus

The TB was first described by Sandifort in 1785 as a RUL bronchus originating from the trachea.[3] Although anatomically incorrect, these defects encompassed a variety of bronchial anomalies originating from the trachea or the main bronchi and directed to the upper lobes territory.[80] An incidence of 0.1% to 2% for right-sided TB and 0.3% to 1% for left-sided TB was reported in bronchographic, bronchoscopic, or CT series.[80–82] Contrary to chest radiography, which

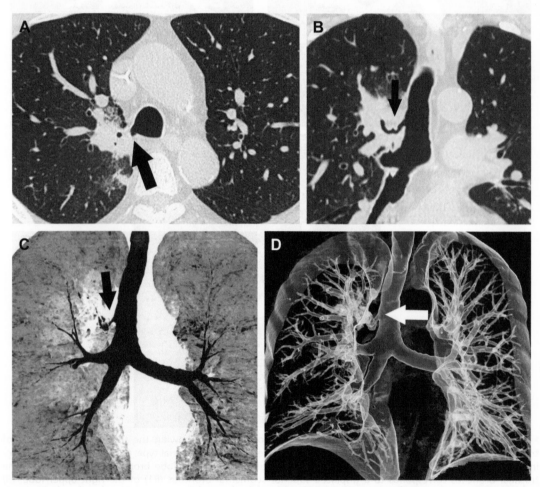

Fig. 7. Displaced and supernumerary right tracheal bronchi. (A–D) Pulmonary infection due to *Streptococcus pneumonia* in the territory ventilated by a supernumerary tracheal bronchus (*arrow*) originating from the trachea (pre-eparterial). The right upper lobe bronchus is displaced on the carina and gives the three modal segmental bronchi. Partial anomalous venous return of right upper pulmonary vein into the superior vena cava is also present (not shown).

demonstrates TB in less than 20% of the patients, chest CT easily diagnoses TB.[15,82,83]

Because in a series of 35 TBs, only 8 originated from the trachea (23%), 3 from the carina (9%), and 24 from more distal bronchi (68%), we use a modified nomenclature from Boyden[84] and Kubik[3] to clarify the classification of aberrant bronchi directed to the upper lobes.[15] The normal RUL bronchus is termed *eparterial* because it arises cranial to the right PA. The normal LUL bronchus is termed *hyparterial* because it arises below the left PA. An anomalous bronchus arising proximal to the origin of the upper lobe bronchus is termed *pre-eparterial* on the right side (**Figs. 6–8**) and *eparterial* or *pre-hyparterial* on the left side (**Fig. 9**). An aberrant bronchus originating distal to the origin of the upper lobe bronchus is termed *post-eparterial* on the right side and *post-hyparterial* on the left side. Double right-sided TBs have been reported.[80,85] Bilateral TBs are found in 6% to 9% of cases (**Fig. 10**).[15,82,86]

A TB is termed *supernumerary* when it coexists with a normal type of branching of the upper lobe bronchus (23%) and *displaced* when, in addition to the aberrant bronchus, one branch of the upper lobe bronchus is missing (77%) (see **Fig. 7**). The displaced type is more frequent than the supernumerary type.[3,15] As Foster-Carter stated, "unless there is a clear evidence that all the normal bronchi are present, as well as the abnormal bronchus, it is always possible that the latter is merely a normal branch arising in an abnormal position (displaced) rather than a true

supernumerary."[70] Bronchial anomalies affecting the upper lobes are seven times more frequent on the right side.[3] The displaced right pre-eparterial bronchus is the most common type (58%). Displaced bronchi ventilate predominantly the apical segment on the right and the apicoposterior segment on the left.[15]

A true TB should designate any bronchus originating from the trachea, usually within 2 cm and up to 6 cm of the carina.[14,82,87] When the entire RUL bronchus is displaced on the trachea, it is called a "pig bronchus" or "bronchus suis;" it has a reported frequency of 0.2% (see **Fig. 6**C).[1,82,83] The angle range of a TB with the trachea is wide and ranges from 22 to 108 degrees (mean, 73 degrees).[82] Occasionally, a TB may ventilate an area of pulmonary tissue separated by its own fissure, which is termed a *tracheal lobe*. An incomplete TB may present as a diverticulum at bronchoscopy (see **Fig. 4**A–C).[88] Vascularization is usually normal for the territory ventilated by the anomalous bronchus.

Although they are usually asymptomatic, recurrent local infections, cough, stridor, acute respiratory distress (especially in children), and hemoptysis can occur if drainage is impaired (narrowing at the TB origin) or if the TB is associated with other abnormalities (see **Figs. 7** and **8**).[80,82,83,85,87,89,90] Clinical symptoms are more frequent in a left-sided TB and in supernumerary TB.[80,81] RUL atelectasis due to endotracheal intubation and even severe hypoxia secondary to TB intubation during anesthesia have been

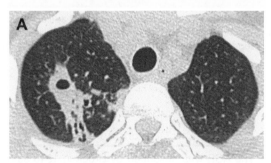
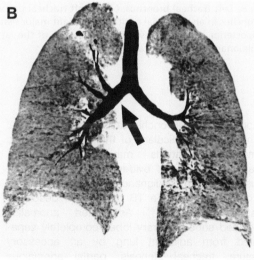

Fig. 8. Tuberculosis and displaced right tracheal bronchus. (*A–B*) Post primary tuberculosis in a territory ventilated by a right tracheal bronchus (B1) arising from right main bronchus (pre-eparterial). Bronchoalveolar lavage was directed into the anomalous bronchus and showed multiresistant mycobacterium tuberculosis that required surgical treatment.

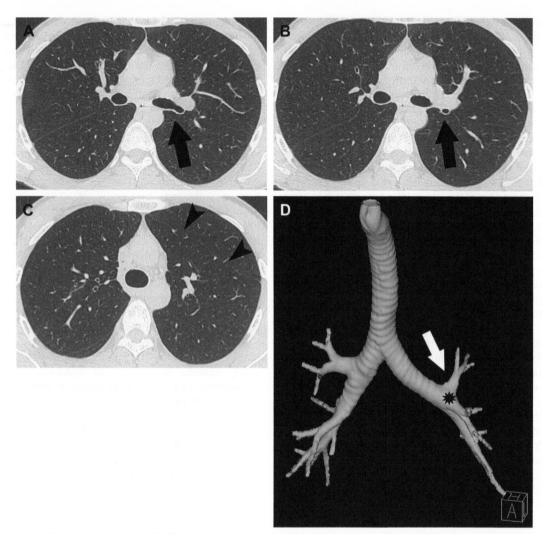

Fig. 9. Left tracheal bronchus. (*A–D*) Left tracheal bronchus (*arrow*) corresponding to a displaced apicoposterior bronchus in an eparterial position. The right major fissure (*arrowheads*) is located between the anterior and apicoposterior segments, resulting in inclusion of the latter segment in the left lower lobe. The level of the left pulmonary artery is indicated by a star.

reported.[82,91,92] Bronchiectasis, atelectasis, focal emphysema (particularly of the LUL), and cystic lung malformations may coexist.[13,80,87,88] Despite the lack of evidence that TB is more susceptible to malignancy, various types of bronchial tumor in a TB have been described as case reports.[93] Associated anomalies included supernumerary lobes completely separated from adjacent lung by an accessory fissure, tracheal stenosis, partial anomalous pulmonary venous return that may drain the abnormal territory, and, uncommonly, congenital heart or other organ diseases.[15,82,87,89]

Accessory Cardiac Bronchus

The ACB was described by Brock in 1946 as the only true supernumerary anomalous bronchus.[94] The reported incidence of ACBs is 0.07% to 0.5%.[15,94–96] The ACB originates from the inner wall of the intermediate bronchus (IB) in 86% of cases and from the RMB in 14%, usually almost opposite to the orifice of the RUL bronchus. Only one ACB originating from the left side has been reported.[97] The abnormal bronchus is demarcated by a spur at its origin in more than 80% of cases. The bronchus has a diameter of 4 to 13.8 mm (mean, 8.7 mm) and advances conically for 5 to

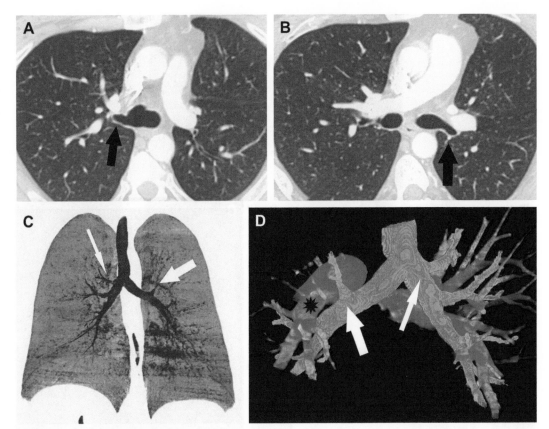

Fig. 10. Bilateral "tracheal" bronchi. (A–D) Right (*long arrows*) and left (*arrows*) tracheal bronchi originate from right and left main bronchi, respectively. The right anomalous bronchus is pre-eparterial and ventilates the superior segment of the right upper lobe (B1). The left is eparterial, as it lies above the arch of the left pulmonary artery (*star*), and ventilates the apicoposterior segment of the left upper lobe (B1+3). The minimum intensity projection reformat is a frontal anterior view and the volume-rendered reformat is a left posterior oblique view.

25 mm (mean, 12 mm) in a caudal direction toward the pericardium, hence the cardiac appellation.[15,96] It is lined by normal bronchial mucosa and has cartilage within its wall, which distinguishes it from an acquired diverticulum, fistula, or adenoid recess. In normal anatomy, the only bronchus arising from the medial wall of the RMB, IB, or RLL bronchus is the paracardiac segmental bronchus (B7). ACB is different from this bronchus which arises from the RLL bronchus and does not correspond to a proximal migration of this structure.[98]

Most ACBs are of the diverticulum type with a blind extremity (71%), but some develop into a series of small bronchioles which may end in a vestigial or rudimentary bronchiolar parenchymal tissue (50%), a ventilated lobulus located in the azygoesophageal recess and demarcated from the RLL by an anomalous fissure (29%), or rarely in cystic degeneration (**Figs. 11** and **12**).[95,96,99,100] An abnormal PA directed to the lobulus has only been reported once.[96]

ACBs are generally asymptomatic and incidentally discovered, but cough, hemoptysis, recurrent infections, empyema, aspergilloma, or even tumor have been reported.[88,95,96,100–102] Surgical resection may be indicated in patients with recurrent or severe symptoms.[102] Associated anomalies include a right- or left-sided TB, coexistence of two ACBs, and bronchiectasis.[15,94,95,100,101]

Bridging Bronchus

A BB is a rarely reported anomaly defined as an anomalous bronchus crossing the midline of the mediastinum from one side to the other, hence the term *bridging*. We found only 25 cases reported as such in the literature up to 2008.[11,62,64–67,103–111]

Two types of BB have been described. In the classic form, the RLL (and sometimes the ML) is ventilated by a bronchus which arises from the medial aspect of the left main bronchus (LMB) and then "bridges" the mediastinum along its

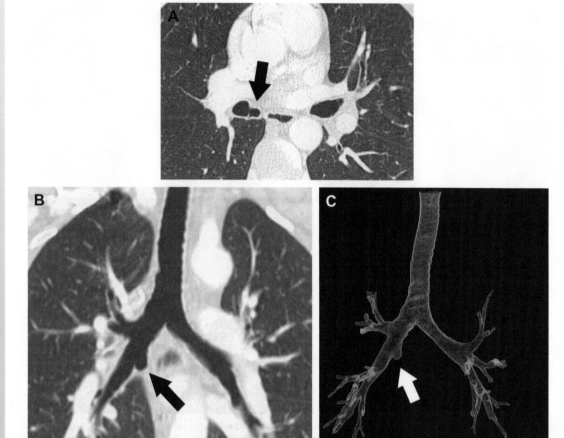

Fig. 11. Accessory cardiac bronchus (diverticulum type). (*A–C*) The blind accessory cardiac bronchus (*arrow*) arises from the medial aspect of the intermediate bronchus as a large-mouthed diverticulum. Curved MPR reformat shows absence of vestigial lung tissue distal to the accessory cardiac bronchus. MPR, multiplanar reformatting.

course to the right lung (**Fig. 13**).[103] In a first subtype of classic BB reported by Holinger in 1950, the RMB is either absent or present only as a short blind tracheal diverticulum at the presumed level of the true carina. This pattern is usually associated with tracheal stenosis and right lung hypoplasia, with the right lung being ventilated only by the BB.[62,106] In a second subtype of classic BB, the trachea is normal in structure and the true carina is located at the normal level, with the RMB ventilating the RUL (and sometimes the ML).[11,103,106,107] Some authors give the denomination of BB to a bronchus located between the true carina and the pseudocarina.[108,110] A second type of BB described only once in the literature is called an "anterior BB." It corresponds to a bronchus originating from the distal anterior aspect of the carina and bridging the mediastinum to the RLL.[109]

The differential diagnosis between the bronchial pattern of a BB and TB may be difficult and remains questionable in some cases (**Fig. 14**).[112,113] Wells and colleagues[65] suggest that the pseudocarina (bifurcation between a BB and LMB) has often been misinterpreted as the true carina; therefore, the RMB is misinterpreted as a TB or pre-eparterial bronchus. Establishing the differential diagnosis between a TB and BB is important because a BB is associated with tracheal and bronchial stenoses due to cartilaginous anomalies, including complete rings, and frequent multiorgan malformations.[11,104] Typically, in normal anatomy, the carina is located at the level of the sixteenth to twentieth cartilaginous rings or the level of T4–T5, and the normal vertical angles for the RMB and LMB are approximately 32 and 50 degrees, respectively.[65] In a BB, the carina (uppermost dichotomy site of the trachea) is located at a normal level, and the

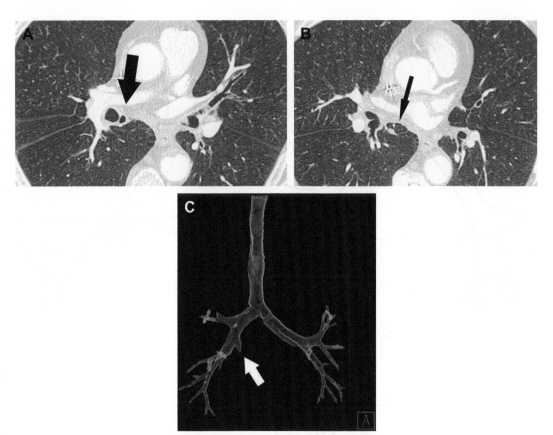

Fig. 12. Accessory cardiac bronchus (with ventilated lobulus). (*A–C*) The accessory cardiac bronchus (*arrow*) originates from the medial wall of the intermediate bronchus and ventilates a small lobulus separated from the right lower lobe by a fissure (*long arrow*).

pseudocarina, corresponding to the site of origin of the BB, is located at the level of T5–T7. The angle is reduced for the proximal LMB (±25 degrees) and normal for the distal LMB below the pseudocarina. The course of the BB is more horizontal (±65 degrees) when compared with the RMB and IB. This difference explains the "inverted T" bronchial pattern seen in the majority of patients with BB, with the angle between the BB and the distal LMB being approximately 115 degrees (see **Fig. 13**).[64,106,107] Furthermore, the pseudocarina is situated substantially to the left of the midline of the trachea.

In most cases, major symptoms consist of respiratory distress and repeated pulmonary infections.[103–105,107] Pulmonary lobes ventilated by a BB can show signs of atelectasis or a cystlike appearance.[103,104] The permanent or iterative poor aeration of the BB lobes may be due to narrowing of the trachea, LMB or BB, compression of the LMB by an SLPA, or kinking or obstruction of the BB secondary to positional changes.[103–105,108,110] The RUL (and ML) may show

hyperinflation that may cause clinical complications such as pneumothorax.[103] In the past, inappropriate surgery on the RUL was performed due to misknowledge of a BB, because the overinflation of the RUL may guide the clinician to a wrong diagnosis of congenital lobar emphysema, bronchial atresia, or overinflation of any acquired cause.[105] A BB should also be differentiated from crossover lung segments and horseshoe lung.[114,115]

Associated thoracic malformations include, among others, vascular anomalies including particularly SLPA,[11,105–108] partial anomalous venous return,[103,104] a bilobate right lung,[103,104] and cardiac or extrathoracic malformations.[66,103,104,106,108]

Other Displaced Bronchi

Minor forms of proximal or distal displacement of segmental or subsegmental bronchi in the same lobe are found in approximately 10% of individuals.[83,84,94] More rarely, a displaced segmental or subsegmental bronchus can originate from an

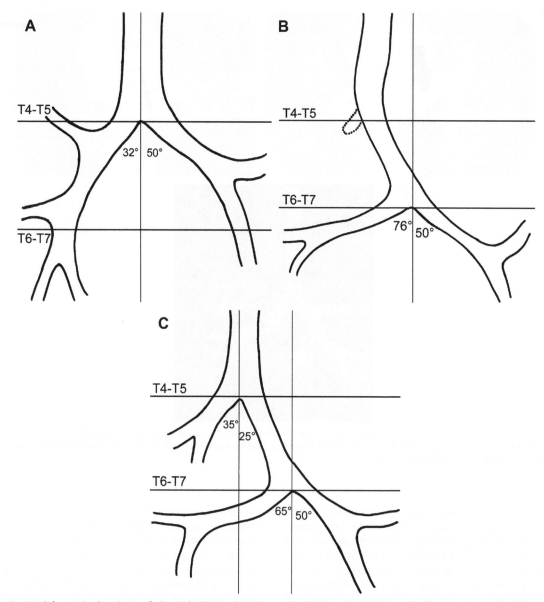

Fig. 13. Schematic drawings of classic bridging bronchus. *(A–C)* Normal anatomy *(A)*, first subtype of bridging bronchus with right upper lobe bronchus presenting as a diverticulum *(B)*, and second subtype of bridging bronchus *(C)*. The level of carina and pseudocarina are indicated. See text for explanations on bronchial angles. *(Courtesy of* Catherine Beigelman, MD, Hopital la Pitie-Salpetriere, Paris, France.)

adjacent lobe.[15] Such variants predominantly involve the upper lobes and particularly the right side.[116] The area ventilated by the displaced bronchus remains normal, but CT often demonstrates a displaced or incomplete fissure between both territories **(Fig. 15)**. The axillary bronchus is one of the most frequently encountered (5%–16%) variants and usually corresponds to a displaced subsegmental bronchus of the posterior or anterior segmental bronchi of the RUL, ventilating the so-called "axillary area" of the RUL **(Fig. 16)**.[94,117,118] Less commonly, the posterior segmental bronchus of the RUL is displaced distally on the IB, which corresponds to a post-hyparterial bronchus in the TB classification (see **Fig. 15**). Occasional displacement or fusion of lobar bronchi is also reported.[3,84] A displaced bronchus responsible for bronchial tangle or interdigitation has been termed a *braided bronchus*.[115]

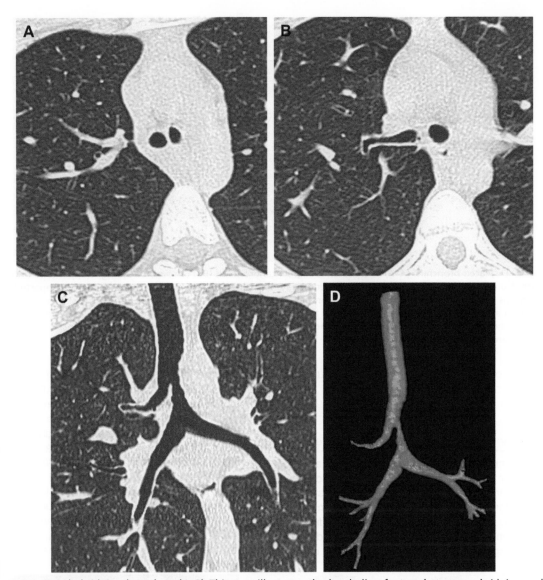

Fig. 14. Pseudo-bridging bronchus. (*A–D*) This case illustrates the borderline feature between a bridging and tracheal bronchus. At a first glance, pro arguments for a bridging bronchus include the general morphologic pattern of the tracheobronchial tree and particularly a stenosis of the "left main bronchus," which may be found in association with such anomalous bronchi. Cons are nevertheless numerous and among others include the finding that the "carina" is located at the level of the aortic arch and "pseudocarina" at the level of T5-T6. The angle of the pseudocarina is that of the true carina and is furthermore not displaced to the left of the midline of the trachea; therefore, this case should be considered as a pseudo-bridging bronchus, namely, a real right tracheal bronchus associated with stenosis of the distal trachea. (*Courtesy of* Catherine Beigelman, MD, Hôpital la Pitié-Salpétrière, Paris, France).

MALFORMATIONS ASSOCIATED WITH ABNORMALITIES OF SITUS

Situs solitus is defined as the modal arrangement of organs and vessels within the body. The right-sided lung is trilobed, and the right atrium is the systemic one receiving blood from the vena cava. On the left side, the lung is bilobed, and the left atrium is the pulmonary one receiving blood from the pulmonary veins. Situs anomalies imply a disordered organ arrangement in the chest and/or abdomen.

Reversal Right–Left, Situs Inversus

Situs inversus is a congenital condition in which the major visceral organs are reversed through the medial sagittal plane from their normal position. It is seen in 0.00005% to 0.01%[119,120] of the

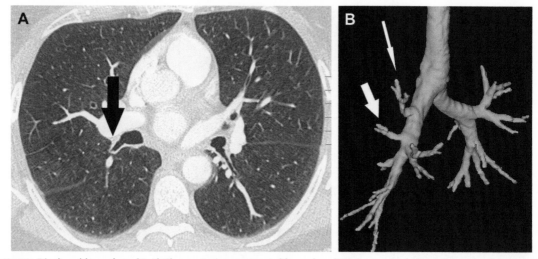

Fig. 15. Displaced bronchus. (*A–B*) The posterior segmental bronchus (B3) (*arrows*) of the right upper lobe originates from the lower posterior part of the intermediate bronchus. This anomaly corresponds to a post-eparterial bronchus in the classification of the tracheal bronchi. The right upper lobe bronchus (*long arrows*) is in its usual location and gives two segmental bronchi for the anterior (B2) and apical segment (B1). The upper part of the right major fissure is posteriorly displaced and incomplete medially. The volume-rendering bronchography is a right anterior oblique view.

population. Kartagener syndrome is found in approximately 20% of patients with situs inversus.[120]

Situs Ambiguous, Heterotaxic Syndromes

Situs ambiguous or heterotaxia refers to anatomic arrangements in which the major organs are dis-tributed abnormally within the chest and/or abdomen. Traditionally, it was common to describe heterotaxic syndromes as the syndromes of asplenia (right isomerism or Ivemark syndrome) or polysplenia (left isomerism). Because of the wide number of possible combinations of malformations and the overlapping spectrum of findings commonly seen, an individualized approach is now preferred describing all malformations present in a particular patient (ie, heterotaxic syndrome of bilateral trilobed lungs, dextrocardia, asplenia, and a left-sided inferior vena cava).[120] When the bronchial tree is involved, the patterns of airways branching and the pulmonary lobation are identical in the two lungs (isomerism), and the structure of both atria is also similar.[120] The thoracic and atrial situs are almost invariably associated, which means, the atrial situs can be determined from

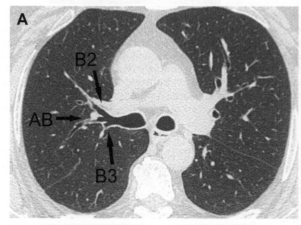
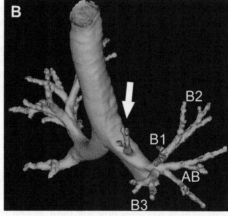

Fig. 16. Axillary bronchus. (*A–B*) Trifurcation pattern of the right upper lobe bronchus in the axial plane with the "axillary bronchus" (AB) ventilating the axillary part of the lobe. Note a supernumerary right tracheal bronchus arising from right main bronchus (*arrow*). B1, superior segmental bronchus; B2, anterior segmental bronchus; B3, posterior segmental bronchus.

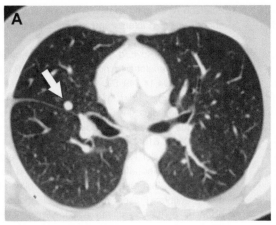
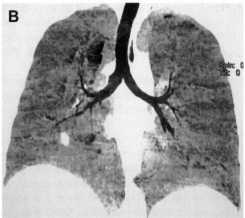

Fig. 17. Left isomerism. (*A–B*) The right lung is smaller than the left one and shows a mirror pattern of left bronchial division (left isomerism). The ratio of the left main bronchus/right main bronchus is 1.17:1. Right lobar bronchi are slightly hypoplastic when compared with the left ones. Right lung also showed a pseudo-scimitar syndrome (meandering vein, *arrow*).

bronchial anatomy.[121,122] According to Partridge and colleagues,[123] a ratio between the length of the LMB and RMB less than 1.5:1 strongly suggests isomerism, with the lowest ratio in situs solitus or inversus being 1.7:1. Nevertheless, exceptional discordances between bronchial and atrial situs have been reported.[123]

In right isomerism or bilateral right-sidedness, the two lungs are trilobed with bilateral minor fissures. The main bronchi are short (<1 cm) and are located superior to the ipsilateral main PA on each side (eparterial bronchi).[121] Both atria are of the systemic type. A left-sided azygos lobe is suggestive of right isomerism.[119,121] Right isomerism is classically associated with asplenia, bilateral systemic atria, a centrally located liver, and a stomach in indeterminate position (Ivemark syndrome). Cardiac anomalies are common (99% to 100%) and complex, and survival beyond 1 year of life is rare, ranging from less than 5% to 20%.[119,120] Right isomerism may rarely exist without cardiac anomalies and exceptionally remain asymptomatic until adulthood (<1%).[119,121]

In left isomerism or bilateral left-sidedness, the lungs are bilobed, minor fissure is absent, and main bronchi are long (1.7–2 cm)[119,121] and hyparterial, passing inferiorly to the ipsilateral main PA on each side (**Fig. 17**). Left isomerism is classically associated with both atria of the pulmonary type, a midline liver, and polysplenia. The location of the stomach is variable. Interruption of the inferior vena cava with azygos or hemiazygos continuation (85%) and anomalous pulmonary venous return are frequently associated.[119,124] Cardiac abnormalities are less common and less complex than

in right isomerism. The death rate is lower, being approximately 60% in the first year of life. Left isomerism may be an incidental finding in an asymptomatic adult, and cases of patients with bilateral bilobed lungs, normal abdominal situs, and the absence of cardiac abnormality have been reported.[119,120,125,126] Left isomerism with bilobed lungs is present in 55% of cases of polysplenia.[119]

SUMMARY

Recognition of bronchial variants and anomalies by the radiologist is an important step in reporting on CT examinations of the chest because it has numerous clinical implications. Precise description is necessary for the pneumologist (for fiberoptic bronchoscopy, bronchoalveolar lavage, biopsy, and endobronchial treatment), the chest surgeon (for lung resection and transplantation), and the anesthesiologist (for endotracheal tube placement).

REFERENCES

1. Lemoine JM, Gagnon A. Principaux modes de division et anomalies anatomiques de la trachée et des bronches. Bronches 1952;2:409–21.
2. Atwell SW. Major anomalies of the tracheobronchial tree, with a list of the minor anomalies. Dis Chest 1967;52:611–5.
3. Kubik S, Müntener M. Bronchusanomalien: tracheale, eparterielle und präeparterielle bronchi. Rofo 1971;114:145–63.
4. Remy J, Remy-Jardin M, Artaud D, et al. Multiplanar and three-dimensional reconstruction techniques in CT: impact on chest diseases. Eur Radiol 1998;8:335–51.

5. Fitoz S, Atasoy C, Yagmurlu A, et al. Three-dimensional CT of congenital esophageal atresia and distal tracheoesophageal fistula in neonates: preliminary results. AJR Am J Roentgenol 2000; 175:1403–7.

6. Kawamoto S, Yuasa M, Tsukuda S, et al. Bronchial atresia: three-dimensional CT bronchography using volume rendering technique. Radiat Med 2001;19: 107–10.

7. Tsuchiya T, Mori K, Ichikawa T, et al. Bronchopulmonary foregut malformation diagnosed by three-dimensional CT. Pediatr Radiol 2003;33:887–9.

8. Siegel MJ. Multiplanar and three-dimensional multidetector row CT of thoracic vessels and airways in the pediatric population. Radiology 2003;229:641–50.

9. Strouse PJ, Newman B, Hernandez RJ, et al. CT of tracheal agenesis. Pediatr Radiol 2006;36:920–6.

10. Heyer CM, Nuesslein TG, Jung D, et al. Tracheobronchial anomalies and stenoses: detection with low-dose multidetector CT with virtual tracheobronchoscopy–comparison with flexible tracheobronchoscopy. Radiology 2007;242:542–9.

11. Baden W, Schaefer J, Kumpf M, et al. Comparison of imaging techniques in the diagnosis of bridging bronchus. Eur Respir J 2008;31:1125–31.

12. Lee EY, Boiselle PM, Cleveland RH. Multidetector CT evaluation of congenital lung anomalies. Radiology 2008;247(3):632–48.

13. Evans JA. Aberrant bronchi and cardiac vascular anomalies. Am J Med Genet 1990;35:46–54.

14. Harris JH Jr. The clinical significance of the tracheal bronchus. AJR Am J Roentgenol 1958; 79:228–34.

15. Ghaye B, Szapiro D, Fanchamps JM, et al. Congenital bronchial abnormalities revisited. Radiographics 2001;21:105–19.

16. Bremer JL. Accessory bronchi in embryos: their occurrence and probable fate. Anat Rec 1932;54: 361–74.

17. Alescio T, Cassini A. Induction in vitro of tracheal buds by pulmonary mesenchyma grafted on tracheal epithelium. J Exp Zool 1962;150:83–94.

18. Merei JM, Hutson JM. Embryogenesis of tracheoesophageal anomalies: a review. Pediatr Surg Int 2002;18(5–6):319–26.

19. Mata JM, Caceres J. The dysmorphic lung: imaging findings. Eur Radiol 1996;6:403–14.

20. Landing BH, Dixon LG. Congenital malformations and genetic disorders of the respiratory tract. Am Rev Respir Dis 1979;20:151–85.

21. Shenoy SS, Culver GJ, Pirson HS. Agenesis of lung in an adult. AJR Am J Roentgenol 1979;133(4): 755–7.

22. Beigelman C, Howarth NR, Chartrand-Lefebvre C, et al. Congenital anomalies of tracheobronchial branching patterns: spiral CT aspects in adults. Eur Radiol 1998;8(1):79–85.

23. Paterson A. Imaging evaluation of congenital lung abnormalities in infants and children. Radiol Clin North Am 2005;43(2):303–23.

24. Woodring JH, Howard TA, Kanga JF. Congenital pulmonary venolobar syndrome revisited. Radiographics 1994;14:349–69.

25. Remy J, Remy-Jardin M. Malformations pulmonaires congénitales. In: Grenier P, editor. Imagerie thoracique de l'adulte. 3rd edition. Paris: Flammarion; 2006. p. 619–58.

26. Fraser RS, Muller NL, Colman N, et al. Developmental anomalies affecting the airways and lung parenchyma. In: Fraser RS, Muller NL, Colman N, et al, editors. Fraser and Paré's diagnosis of diseases of the chest. 4th edition. Philadelphia: WB Saunders; 1999. p. 597–635.

27. Gerle RD, Jaretzki A 3rd, Ashley CA, et al. Congenital bronchopulmonary-foregut malformation: pulmonary sequestration communicating with the gastrointestinal tract. N Engl J Med 1968;278:1413–9.

28. Heithoff KB, Sane SM, Williams HJ, et al. Bronchopulmonary foregut malformations: a unifying etiological concept. AJR Am J Roentgenol 1976;126: 46–55.

29. Osinowo O, Harley HR, Janigan D. Congenital broncho-oesophageal fistula in the adult. Thorax 1983;38:138–42.

30. Leithiser RE Jr, Capitanio MA, Macpherson RI, et al. "Communicating" bronchopulmonary foregut malformations. AJR Am J Roentgenol 1986;146: 227–31.

31. Srikanth MS, Ford EG, Stanley P, et al. Communicating bronchopulmonary foregut malformations: classification and embryogenesis. J Pediatr Surg 1992;27:732–6.

32. Verma A, Mohan S, Kathuria M, et al. Esophageal bronchus: case report and review of the literature. Acta Radiol 2008;49:138–41.

33. Keeley JL, Schairer AE. The anomalous origin of the right main bronchus from the esophagus. Ann Surg 1960;152:871–4.

34. Tsugawa J, Tsugawa C, Satoh S, et al. Communicating bronchopulmonary foregut malformation: particular emphasis on concomitant congenital tracheobronchial stenosis. Pediatr Surg Int 2005; 21:932–5.

35. Lacina S, Townley R, Radecki L, et al. Esophageal lung with cardiac abnormalities. Chest 1981;79: 468–70.

36. Lallemand D, Quignodon JF, Courtel JV. The anomalous origin of bronchus from the esophagus: report of three cases. Pediatr Radiol 1996;26: 179–82.

37. Singal AK, Kumar VR, Rao M, et al. Bilateral communicating bronchopulmonary foregut malformations in a child. Ann Thorac Surg 2006;82: 330–2.

38. Braimbridge MV, Keith HI. Oesophago-bronchial fistula in the adult. Thorax 1965;20:226–33.

39. Risher WH, Arensman RM, Ochsner JL. Congenital bronchoesophageal fistula. Ann Thorac Surg 1990; 49:500–5.

40. Im JG, Lee WJ, Han MC, et al. Congenital broncho-oesophageal fistula in the adult. Clin Radiol 1991; 43:380–4.

41. Nagata K, Kamio Y, Ichikawa T, et al. Congenital tracheoesophageal fistula successfully diagnosed by CT esophagography. World J Gastroenterol 2006;12:1476–8.

42. Sumner TE, Auringer ST, Cox TD. A complex communicating bronchopulmonary foregut malformation: diagnostic imaging and pathogenesis. Pediatr Radiol 1997;27:799–801.

43. Islam S, Cavanaugh E, Honeke R, et al. Diagnosis of a proximal tracheoesophageal fistula using three-dimensional CT scan: a case report. J Pediatr Surg 2004;39:100–2.

44. Sandu K, Monnier P. Congenital tracheal anomalies. Otolaryngol Clin North Am 2007;40:193–217.

45. Floyd J, Campbell DC Jr, Dominy DE. Agenesis of the trachea. Am Rev Respir Dis 1962;86:557–60.

46. Ramsay BH, Byron FX. Mucocele, congenital bronchiectasis, and bronchiogenic cyst. J Thorac Surg 1953;26:21–30.

47. Remy J, Ribet M, Pagniez B, et al. [Segmentary bronchial atresia: study of 3 cases and review of the literature]. Ann Radiol 1973;16:615–28.

48. Jederlinic PJ, Sicilian LS, Baigelman W, et al. Congenital bronchial atresia: a report of 4 cases and a review of the literature. Medicine 1986;65:73–83.

49. Ward S, Morcos SK. Congenital bronchial atresia: presentation of three cases and a pictorial review. Clin Radiol 1999;54:144–8.

50. Matsushima H, Takayanagi N, Satoh M, et al. Congenital bronchial atresia: radiologic findings in nine patients. J Comput Assist Tomogr 2002;26:860–4.

51. Seo T, Ando H, Kaneko K, et al. Two cases of prenatally diagnosed congenital lobar emphysema caused by lobar bronchial atresia. J Pediatr Surg 2006;41:e17–20.

52. Kinsella D, Sissons G, Williams MP. The radiological imaging of bronchial atresia. Br J Radiol 1992;65:681–5.

53. Berrocal T, Madrid C, Novo S, et al. Congenital anomalies of the tracheobronchial tree, lung, and mediastinum: embryology, radiology, and pathology. Radiographics 2004;24(1):e17.

54. Pedicelli G, Ciarpaglini LL, De Santis M, et al. Congenital bronchial atresia (CBA): a critical review of CBA as a disease entity and presentation of a case series. Radiol Med 2005;110:544–53.

55. Morikawa N, Kuroda T, Honna T, et al. Congenital bronchial atresia in infants and children. J Pediatr Surg 2005;40:1822–6.

56. Ko SF, Lee TY, Kao CL, et al. Bronchial atresia associated with epibronchial right pulmonary artery and aberrant right middle lobe artery. Br J Radiol 1998;71:217–20.

57. Cohen AM, Solomon EH, Alfidi RJ. Computed tomography in bronchial atresia. AJR Am J Roentgenol 1980;135:1097–9.

58. Okuda M, Huang CL, Masuya D, et al. Lobar bronchial atresia demonstrating a cystic lesion without overinflation. Eur J Cardiothorac Surg 2006;30:391–3.

59. Agarwal PP, Matzinger FR, Seely JM, et al. An unusual case of systemic arterial supply to the lung with bronchial atresia. AJR Am J Roentgenol 2005;185:150–3.

60. Yoon YH, Son KH, Kim JT, et al. Bronchial atresia associated with spontaneous pneumothorax: report of a case. J Korean Med Sci 2004;19:142–4.

61. Kunisaki SM, Fauza DO, Nemes LP, et al. Bronchial atresia: the hidden pathology within a spectrum of prenatally diagnosed lung masses. J Pediatr Surg 2006;41:61–5.

62. Holinger PH, Johnston KC, Basinger CE. Benign stenosis of the trachea. Ann Otol Rhinol Laryngol 1950;59:837–59.

63. Chang N, Hertzler JH, Gregg RH, et al. Congenital stenosis of the right mainstem bronchus: a case report. Pediatrics 1968;41:739–42.

64. Berdon WE, Baker DH, Wung JT, et al. Complete cartilage-ring tracheal stenosis associated with anomalous left pulmonary artery: the ring-sling complex. Radiology 1984;152:57–64.

65. Wells TR, Gwinn JL, Landing BH, et al. Reconsideration of the anatomy of sling left pulmonary artery: the association of one form with bridging bronchus and imperforate anus. Anatomic and diagnostic aspects. J Pediatr Surg 1988;23:892–8.

66. Lee KH, Yoon CS, Choe KO, et al. Use of imaging for assessing anatomical relationships of tracheobronchial anomalies associated with left pulmonary artery sling. Pediatr Radiol 2001;31:269–78.

67. Berdon WE. Rings, slings, and other things: vascular compression of the infant trachea updated from the midcentury to the millennium–the legacy of Robert E. Gross, MD, and Edward B.D. Neuhauser, MD. Radiology 2000;216:624–32.

68. Foster-Carter AF. Broncho-pulmonary abnormalities. Br J Tuberc Dis Chest 1946;40:111–24.

69. Woodring JH, Howard RS 2nd, Rehm SR. Congenital tracheobronchomegaly (Mounier-Kuhn syndrome): a report of 10 cases and review of the literature. J Thorac Imaging 1991;6(2):1–10.

70. Frenkiel S, Assimes IK, Rosales JK. Congenital tracheal diverticulum: a case report. Ann Otol Rhinol Laryngol 1980;89:406–8.

71. Early EK, Bothwell MR. Congenital tracheal diverticulum. Otolaryngol Head Neck Surg 2002; 127(1):119–21.

72. Caversaccio MD, Becker M, Zbären P. Tracheal diverticulum presenting with recurrent laryngeal nerve paralysis. Ann Otol Rhinol Laryngol 1998; 107(4):362–4.

73. Restrepo S, Villamil MA, Rojas IC, et al. Association of two respiratory congenital anomalies: tracheal diverticulum and cystic adenomatoid malformation of the lung. Pediatr Radiol 2004;34(3):263–6.

74. Goo JM, Im JG, Ahn JM, et al. Right paratracheal air cysts in the thoracic inlet: clinical and radiologic significance. AJR Am J Roentgenol 1999;173(1):65–70.

75. Soto-Hurtado EJ, Peñuela-Ruíz L, Rivera-Sánchez I, et al. Tracheal diverticulum: a review of the literature. Lung 2006;184(6):303–7.

76. McKinnon D. Tracheal diverticula. J Pathol Bacteriol 1953;65:513–7.

77. Polverosi R, Carloni A, Poletti V. Tracheal and main bronchial diverticula: the role of CT. Radiol Med 2008;113(2):181–9.

78. Sanford MF, Broderick LS. Multidetector computed tomography detection of bronchial diverticula. J Thorac Imaging 2007;22:265–7.

79. Koffi-Aka V, Manceau A, Cottier JP, et al. [Tracheocele: a rare cause of pharyngeal disorders]. Ann Otolaryngol Chir Cervicofac 2002;119(3):186–8.

80. Ming Z, Lin Z. Evaluation of tracheal bronchus in Chinese children using multidetector CT. Pediatr Radiol 2007;37:1230–4.

81. Remy J, Smith M, Marache P, et al. La bronche "trachéale" gauche pathogène. J Radiol Electrol 1977; 58:621–30.

82. Ritsema GH. Ectopic right bronchus: indications for bronchography. AJR Am J Roentgenol 1983;140: 671–4.

83. Feofilov GL, Ossipov VP. Bronche trachéale. Bronches 1970;20:274–83.

84. Boyden EA. Segmental anatomy of the lungs. New York: McGraw-Hill; 1995.

85. Iannaccone G, Capocaccia P, Colloridi V, et al. Double right tracheal bronchus: a case report in an infant. Pediatr Radiol 1983;13:156–8.

86. Kumagae Y, Jinguji M, Tanaka D, et al. An adult case of bilateral true tracheal bronchi associated with hemoptysis. J Thorac Imaging 2006;21:293–5.

87. Siegel MJ, Shackelford GD, Francis RS, et al. Tracheal bronchus. Radiology 1979;130:353–5.

88. Yildiz H, Ugurel S, Soylu K, et al. Accessory cardiac bronchus and tracheal bronchus anomalies: CT-bronchoscopy and CT-bronchography findings. Surg Radiol Anat 2006;28:646–9.

89. McLaughlin FJ, Strieder DJ, Harris GBC, et al. Tracheal bronchus: association with respiratory morbidity in childhood. J Pediatr 1985;106:751–5.

90. Middleton RM, Littleton JT, Brickey DA, et al. Obstructed tracheal bronchus as a cause of postobstructive pneumonia. J Thorac Imaging 1995; 10:223–4.

91. Stene R, Rose M, Weinger MB, et al. Bronchial trifurcation at the carina complicating use of a double-lumen tracheal tube. Anesthesiology 1994;80:1162–4.

92. O'Sullivan BP, Frassica JJ, Rayder SM. Tracheal bronchus: a cause of prolonged atelectasis in intubated children. Chest 1998;113:537–40.

93. Patrinou V, Kourea H, Dougenis D. Bronchial carcinoid of an accessory tracheal bronchus. Ann Thorac Surg 2001;71:1034–5.

94. Brock RC. The anatomy of the bronchial tree. London: Oxford University Press; 1946.

95. Mangiulea VG, Stinghe RV. The accessory cardiac bronchus: bronchologic aspect and review of the literature. Dis Chest 1968;54:35–8.

96. Ghaye B, Kos X, Dondelinger RF. Accessory cardiac bronchus: 3D CT demonstration in nine cases. Eur Radiol 1999;9:45–8.

97. Lachowicz D, Trzebińska-Korniszewska A. [Unusual left-side bronchial anomaly]. Rofo 1978; 129(2):271–2.

98. Ghaye B. Accessory cardiac bronchus. Radiographics 2000;20:1493.

99. Huzly A, Boehm F. Bronches cardiaques accessoires. Bronches 1956;6:540–50.

100. McGuinness G, Naidich DP, Garay SM, et al. Accessory cardiac bronchus: CT features and clinical significance. Radiology 1993;189:563–6.

101. Jackson GD, Littleton JT. Simultaneous occurrence of anomalous cardiac and tracheal bronchi: a case report. J Thorac Imaging 1988;3:59–60.

102. Bentala M, Grijm K, van der Zee JH, et al. Cardiac bronchus: a rare cause of hemoptysis. Eur J Cardiothorac Surg 2002;22:643–5.

103. Gonzalez-Crussi F, Padilla LM, Miller JK, et al. Bridging bronchus: a previously undescribed airway anomaly. Am J Dis Child 1976;130:1015–8.

104. Starshak RJ, Sty JR, Woods G, et al. Bridging bronchus: a rare airway anomaly. Radiology 1981;140:95–6.

105. Bertucci GM, Dickman PS, Lachman RS, et al. Bridging bronchus and posterior left pulmonary artery: a unique association. Pediatr Pathol 1987; 7:637–43.

106. Wells TR, Stanley P, Padua EM, et al. Serial section-reconstruction of anomalous tracheobronchial branching patterns from CT scan images: bridging bronchus associated with sling left pulmonary artery. Pediatr Radiol 1990;20:444–6.

107. Stokes JR, Heatley DG, Lusk RP, et al. The bridging bronchus: successful diagnosis and repair. Arch Otolaryngol Head Neck Surg 1997;123:1344–7.

108. Grillo HC, Wright CD, Vlahakes GJ, et al. Management of congenital tracheal stenosis by means of slide tracheoplasty or resection and reconstruction, with long-term follow-up of growth after slide tracheoplasty. J Thorac Cardiovasc Surg 2002; 123(1):145–52.

109. Rishavy TJ, Goretsky MJ, Langenburg SE, et al. Anterior bridging bronchus. Pediatr Pulmonol 2003;35:70–2.

110. Topcu S, Liman ST, Sarisoy HT, et al. Stenotic bridging bronchus: a very rare entity. J Thorac Cardiovasc Surg 2006;131:1200–1.

111. Lee ML, Lue HC, Chiu IS, et al. A systematic classification of the congenital bronchopulmonary vascular malformations: dysmorphogeneses of the primitive foregut system and the primitive aortic arch system. Yonsei Med J 2008;49:90–102.

112. Gower WA, McGrath-Morrow SA, MacDonald KD, et al. Tracheal bronchus in a 6-month-old infant identified by CT with three-dimensional airway reconstruction. Thorax 2008;63:93–4.

113. Cope R, Campbell JR, Wall M. Bilateral tracheal bronchi. J Pediatr Surg 1986;21(5):443–4.

114. Clements BS, Warner JO. The crossover lung segment: congenital malformation associated with a variant of scimitar syndrome. Thorax 1987;42:417–9.

115. Wheeler DS, Poss WB, Cocalis M, et al. Braided bronchus: a previously undescribed airway anomaly. Pediatr Pulmonol 1998;25:348–51.

116. Odell J. Anomalous origin of the anterior segmental bronchus of the right upper lobe. Thorax 1980;35:213–4.

117. Wu JW, White CS, Meyer CA, et al. Variant bronchial anatomy: CT appearance and classification. AJR Am J Roentgenol 1999;172:741–4.

118. MacGregor JH, Chiles C, Godwin JD, et al. Imaging of the axillary subsegment of the right upper lobe. Chest 1986;90(5):763–5.

119. Winer-Muram HT. Adult presentation of heterotaxic syndromes and related complexes. J Thorac Imaging 1995;10(1):43–57.

120. Applegate KE, Goske MJ, Pierce G, et al. Situs revisited: imaging of the heterotaxy syndrome. Radiographics 1999;19(4):837–52.

121. Winer-Muram HT, Tonkin IL. The spectrum of heterotaxic syndromes. Radiol Clin North Am 1989;27(6):1147–70.

122. Bush A. Left bronchial isomerism, normal atrial arrangement and bronchomalacia mimicking asthma: a new syndrome? Eur Respir J 1999;14(2):475–7.

123. Partridge JB, Scott O, Deverall PB, et al. Visualization and measurement of the main bronchi by tomography as an objective indicator of thoracic situs in congenital heart disease. Circulation 1975;51:188–96.

124. Ruscazio M, Van Praagh S, Marrass AR, et al. Interrupted inferior vena cava in asplenia syndrome and a review of the hereditary patterns of visceral situs abnormalities. Am J Cardiol 1998;81(1):111–6.

125. Winer-Muram H, Ellis JV, Scott RL, et al. Isolated left thoracic isomerism. Radiology 1985;155:10.

126. Landay MJ, Chaw C, Bordlee RP. Bilateral left lungs: unusual variation of hilar anatomy. AJR Am J Roentgenol 1982;138:1162–4.

Imaging of Tumors of the Trachea and Central Bronchi

G.R. Ferretti, MD, PhD[a,b,c,*], C. Bithigoffer, MD[b],
C.A. Righini, MD, PhD[b,c,d], F. Arbib, MD[e],
S. Lantuejoul, MD, PhD[b,c,f], A. Jankowski, MD[b]

KEYWORDS
- CT • Chest radiography • Trachea
- Main bronchi • Malignant tumor • Benign tumor

Primary tumors of the trachea and main bronchi are rare, accounting for 1% to 2% of all respiratory tract tumors.[1,2] In adults, most (60%–90%) of these tumors are malignant,[3,4] whereas benign tumors represent the majority of lesions in children. Among those tumors in adults, squamous cell carcinoma (SCC) and adenoid cystic carcinoma (ACC) are the most frequent, representing approximately 80% of all tumors of the trachea and main bronchi. Other tumors are less common, arising from epithelial or mesenchymal tissue, and constitute a large list of heterogeneous benign and malignant tumors (**Table 1**). Imaging plays a key role in depicting these tumors and assessing tumor extent within the lumen, airway wall, and surrounding structures before treatment planning.[2,5] Multidetector computed tomography (MDCT) has increased the quality of noninvasive imaging with the recent introduction of isotropic resolution and high quality two- and three-dimensional postprocessing.[6,7] Despite the high quality of CT, there is considerable overlap in CT appearance of most tumors; histologic evaluation is needed in nearly all cases.

CLINICAL PRESENTATION

Centrally located tumors of the airways present with a limited number of signs and symptoms generally related to the obstruction of the airways (eg, dyspnea, acute respiratory failure, wheezing, stridor, recurrent pneumonia, bronchiectasis, atelectasis), whereas other symptoms are not specific (eg, cough, expectoration, hemoptysis).[3] Clinical findings may erroneously suggest the presence of asthma or chronic obstructive lung disease.[1] In other cases, these tumors may be asymptomatic and the lesions are discovered incidentally. The mean duration of symptoms is shorter in patients with malignant tumors (4 months) compared to patients with benign neoplasms (8 months), with the exception of patients with ACCs (12 months).[3]

MULTIDETECTOR COMPUTED TOMOGRAPHY TECHNIQUE

MDCT technology has completely modified the diagnostic approach and the noninvasive planning of treatment in patients who present with central

[a] Clinique Universitaire de Radiologie et Imagerie Médicale, CHU Grenoble, 38043 Grenoble cedex, France
[b] Université J Fourier, Clinique Universitaire de Radiologie et Imagerie Médicale, CHU Grenoble, 38043 Grenoble cedex, France
[c] INSERM U 823, Institut A Bonniot, la Tronche, France
[d] Clinique ORL, CHU Grenoble, 38043 Grenoble cedex, France
[e] Clinique de Pneumologie, CHU Grenoble, 38043 Grenoble cedex, France
[f] Pôle de biologie-Département d'Anatomie et Cytologie Pathologiques, CHU Grenoble, 38043 Grenoble cedex, France
* Corresponding author. Clinique universitaire de radiologie et imagerie médicale, CHU Grenoble, 38043 Grenoble cedex, France.
E-mail address: gferretti@chu-grenoble.fr (G.R. Ferretti).

Radiol Clin N Am 47 (2009) 227–241
doi:10.1016/j.rcl.2008.11.010

Table 1
Classification of tracheal tumors

Epithelial Neoplasms	Mesenchymal Neoplasms
Surface epithelium	
Malignant	*Malignant*
SCC	Soft-tissue sarcomas
Adenocarcinoma	Chondrosarcoma
Large cell carcinoma	Lymphomas
Neuroendocrine tumors	*Benign*
Carcinoids (typical and atypical)	Lipoma
Large cell neuroendocrine tumor	Fibroma
Small cell carcinoma	Fibromatosis
Benign	Histiocytoma
Papilloma	Hemangioma
Papillomatosis	Hemangiopericytoma
	Chemodectoma
Salivary glands	Leiomyoma
Malignant	Granular cell tumor
Adenoid cystic carcinoma	Schwann cell tumors
Mucoepidermoid carcinoma	Chondroma
Carcinoma	Chondroblastoma
Benign	Secondary tumors
Adenoma, pleiomorphic	Invasion by adjacent malignancy (esophagus, thyroid, larynx, lung); hematogenous metastases
Adenoma, mucous gland	
Myoepithelioma	
Onconcytoma	

airway neoplasms.[6] Currently, MDCT enables acquisition of overlapped (30%–50%) thin section (< 1 mm) images with voxels of almost cubic dimensions (isotropic resolution) of the entire airways in a single apnea of few seconds. Fast gantry rotation (< 0.5 seconds) increases the temporal resolution of CT images. Contrast media administration is usually needed to analyze the relationships of tumors of the central airways with the surrounding anatomy and evaluate the contrast enhancement of the tumor. We typically inject 90 to 110 mL of nonionic contrast medium at a rate of 3 mL/s through a peripheral catheter. The natural high contrast between the airways and their environment allows reduction of radiation dose (80–120 kV, 70–160 mAs), particularly in children and young adults. Data should be reconstructed with a high spatial resolution kernel and a soft-tissue resolution kernel. Acquisition is usually performed at full inspiration but can be performed at the end of expiration or during expiration to study the dynamic of the airways and the impact of a tumor on the distal airways and lung parenchyma.[8] With isotropic images, the spatial resolution of images in any reformatted plane is equivalent to the resolution in the transaxial plane, which allows for the creation of excellent two- and three-dimensional reformatted images.[6]

POSTPROCESSING OF CT DATA

Postprocessing offers the opportunity to visualize the trachea and bronchi along their main axis, on external three-dimensional views, or on internal bronchoscopic images.[8–11] Multiplanar reformations in sagittal, coronal, or oblique planes create planar images that eliminate the known limitations of axial images, that is, the partial ability to detect subtle airway stenoses, the underestimation of longitudinal extent of narrowing, the inadequate representation of the airways oriented obliquely to axial plane, and the difficulty to display complex three-dimensional anatomy of the airways.[10] Adding high-quality three-dimensional reconstructions—whether the representation of the air cast[8] or the endoluminal view using virtual bronchoscopy (VB)[7,12]—may even enhance the detection of localized or diffuse diseases.

Three-dimensional surface rendering selects the surface of the column of air contained in the airways by thresholding. Most initial data are lost in the final reconstruction. Shading the surface creates the impression of depth. Although this technique offers an overview of the disease and allows for better understanding of extent of airway narrowing, it suffers from limitations, mainly because of the choice of threshold, which may artificially increase or decrease the size of airways.[6] With volume-rendering techniques, all the information contained in data acquisition is used in the final three-dimensional images. External three-dimensional volume rendering of the airways shows the surface of the airways and the adjacent anatomy, creating CT bronchographic images.[13] Such images enhance the detection of mild airway stenoses.[14]

Burke and colleagues[15] showed an excellent correlation between VB and conventional bronchoscopy regarding the description of stenotic shape and contour and stenosis-to-lumen ratio. Sensitivity of VB was 100% for detection of obstructive bronchogenic carcinoma and 83% for endoluminal nonobstructive neoplasms but 0% for mucosal abnormalities.[16] VB allows passing through high-grade airway stenosis to assess distal airways, which is impossible using classic bronchoscopy.[17] VB can provide a road map for bronchoscopy and guide transbronchial biopsy.[18] Main limitations of VB include false-positive results related to mucus or coagulated blood pseudotumors and the inability to visualize the mucosa or perform biopsy.

Thin slab maximum intensity projection should not be used to detect or characterize airway stenosis because selection of high-density voxels artificially increases the severity of stenosis in eliminating air-containing voxels and may even create artificial stenosis.[8] On the other hand, thin slab minimum intensity projection may artificially decrease the size of asymmetrical narrowing by specifically selecting air-containing voxels. Intraluminal growth of eccentric tumors is underestimated and may be completely ignored.[8] Viewing two- and three-dimensional images simultaneously on a workstation is beneficial for radiologists in increasing their diagnostic ability and confidence in their findings.[19] Two- and three-dimensional images facilitate the communication of information to colleagues who are not familiar with axial anatomy and improve preoperative planning of surgery and bronchoscopy and postprocedural noninvasive evaluation.[20]

CT BRONCHOSCOPIC CORRELATIONS

Lesions larger than 5 mm within the airways are usually detected using CT because of the excellent natural contrast between luminal air and soft-tissue density of lesions. Limitations of MDCT are well known: lesions smaller than 2 to 3 mm are not detected, whereas subtle irregularities of airway walls often result from prominent bronchial cartilage or volume averaging. CT is not able to separate between mucosal and submucosal lesions.

CLASSIFICATION OF MAIN AIRWAYS STENOSES

Surgery is the optimal therapy for malignant and benign tumors of central airways.[1,3,21] Radiation therapy is an option, as is endoluminal therapy.[4] MDCT is useful for detecting, describing, and grading airway stenosis. Description of the lesion should mention the precise location of the tumor, the distance from the cricoid cartilage to the upper limit of the tumor, the distance from the lower part of the lesion to the carina, and the craniocaudal length and its relationship to surrounding structures, including mediastinal vessels and esophagus. Using the same acquisition, enlarged lymph nodes, pulmonary metastases, and postobstructive complications can be described.

In order to standardize the therapeutic approach of airways stenoses, Freitag and colleagues[22] proposed a new classification system. This classification identified twp groups of airway stenoses (structural and dynamic); each structural stenosis is described according to the following categories:

1. *The type of the stenosis.* Type I: exophitic intraluminal tumor or granulation tissue; type II: extrinsic compression; type III: distortion, kinking, bending, or buckling; type IV: scarring or shrinking.
2. *The degree of stenosis* (0%, approximately 25%, approximately 50%, approximately 75%, approximately 90%, complete occlusion).
3. *The location of the stenosis.* Location I: upper third of the trachea; location II: middle third of the trachea; location III: lower third of the trachea; location IV: right main bronchus; location V: left main bronchus.
4. *The transition zone.* The transition zone or the abruptness of stenosis is relevant for treatment planning.

Most tumors of the trachea and main bronchi are type 1. Radiologists may use this classification in their reports to simplify communication with interventional pulmonologists, otorhinolaryngologists, or thoracic surgeons.

MALIGNANT TUMORS

Primary tracheal cancer is rare and its incidence is low compared to laryngeal or bronchial cancer.

It accounts for approximately 0.2% of malignant neoplasms of the respiratory tract.[21] It is more common in men in their 60s with a history of smoking. The prognosis of patients is poor, with the 5-year survival rate being 5% to 35%.[21] The distribution of histologic types of neoplasms may vary regarding the origin of data (surgical versus medical series). In surgical series, SCC accounts for approximately 50% of cases, ACC for approximately 30%, and carcinoid for approximately 10%.[3] The national Danish Cancer registry report (1978–1995) showed that SCC accounted for 63% of tracheal cancers and ACC for only 7% of cases.[23]

SQUAMOUS CELL CARCINOMA

SCC is the most frequent primary malignancy of the trachea, affecting predominantly men (sex ratio 4:1) between age 50 and 60. SCC is strongly associated with cigarette smoking and consequently with other smoking-related cancers of the upper and lower respiratory tract.[1] Macroscopically, SCC appears as a large mass within the central airways with either exophytic or ulcerative component. It can be multifocal in approximately 10% of patients. Regional extent into the esophagus or mainstem bronchi is frequent. The tumor often spreads to regional lymph nodes.

Chest radiography in patients with SCC is often considered unremarkable, but retrospective analysis usually shows focalized asymmetrical filling defect within the tracheal lumen. CT demonstrates a polypoid intraluminal mass of soft tissue density with irregular, smooth, or lobulated contours (**Fig. 1**).[2] The relationships of the tumor with the tracheal wall vary from localized eccentric pedunculated lesions to circumferential invasion. CT shows the extent to the adjacent anatomy. In some patients, the extent of SCC to the esophagus results in tracheoesophageal or bronchoesophageal fistulization.

ADENOID CYSTIC CARCINOMA

ACC is a low-grade malignancy formerly named cylindroma that is not associated with cigarette smoking.[21] It occurs in patients in their 40s; there is no sex predilection. ACC arises from the epithelium of the glands lining the mucosa of the airways and is the most common tumor of the mucosal glands. (It is also named sialadenoid tumor.)[24] In the central airways, ACC has a propensity to infiltrate the wall of the airways and spread along submucosal and perineural planes.[25] ACC grows slowly and is rarely associated with regional lymph node metastases. Distant metastases are rare and often are diagnosed late after the ACC but may present an intense fluorodeoxyglucose uptake.[26] Despite nonspecific signs or symptoms, early recognition of ACC may improve the surgical resectability and the prognosis of patients. Most of the tumors arise in the lower trachea or mainstem bronchi.

Unfortunately, chest radiography is often considered unremarkable; however, an intraluminal mass with smooth, irregular, or lobulated margins can be identified. CT shows a well-limited soft-tissue attenuating intraluminal mass that often infiltrates the airway wall (**Fig. 2**) and the surrounding mediastinal fat.[25] Other presentations include circumferential wall thickening of the trachea creating localized stenosis (**Fig. 3**) or multifocal narrowing.

MUCOEPIDERMOID CARCINOMA

This rare tumor originates from the minor salivary glands lining the tracheobronchial tree.[27] It usually occurs in patients younger than age 40 and affects

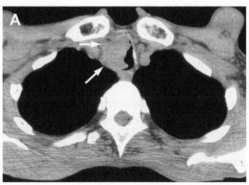
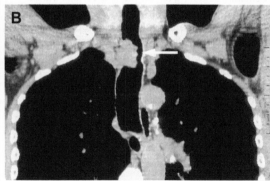

Fig. 1. Squamous cell carcinoma in a 63-year-old man. (*A*) Axial CT at the level of the upper trachea shows a lobulated, intraluminal mass extending to the cartilages of the trachea and to the mediastinal fat (*arrow*). (*B*) Coronal reformation of CT data shows the longitudinal extent of the tumor and the severity of the asymmetrical narrowing of the tracheal lumen (*arrow*).

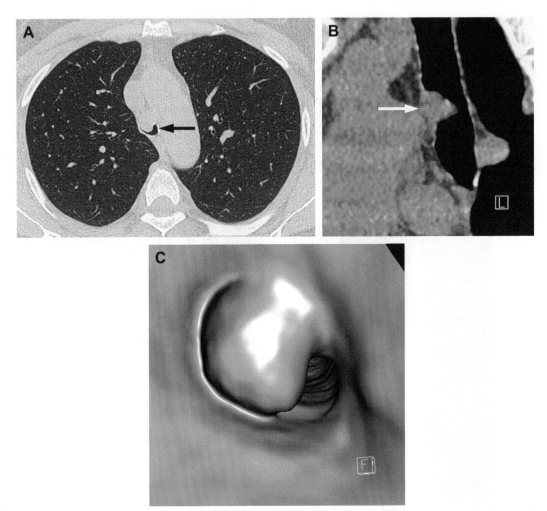

Fig. 2. Adenoid cystic carcinoma in a 36-year-old patient with clinical history of asthma. (A) Axial CT at the level of the aortic arch demonstrates severe narrowing of the lower trachea (arrow). (B) Sagittal reformation shows the large pedicle of the tumor and extraluminal component of the tumor (arrow). (C) Virtual endoscopy demonstrates the severity of the tracheal stenosis.

mainly the segmental bronchi,[28] creating airway obstruction. It is even rarer than ACC, representing 5% of sialadenoid tumors. Histologicaly, mucoepidermoid carcinoma associates variable proportions of squamous cells, mucus secreting cells, and intermediate cells with variable degree of mitoses, nuclear pleomorphism, and cellular necrosis, defining low- or high-grade malignancy (Fig. 4).[28]

Mucoepidermoid carcinoma shows the same CT pattern as bronchial carcinoid tumors. It presents as an endobronchial mass, often smoothly oval or lobulated with its long axis parallel to that of the airways containing the tumor, but contrast enhancement is usually mild.[28] Punctate calcifications within the tumor were present in 6 of 12 cases.[28] CT contrast enhancement of mucoepidermoid carcinoma has been differently

appreciated: mild enhancement was reported by Kim and colleagues,[28] whereas marked heterogeneous contrast enhancement was reported in four of five cases in a small series by Ishizumi and colleagues.[29] The presence of abundant microvessels at histopathology correlated with the CT findings.[29] Lymphadenopathy is rare.

CARCINOID TUMORS

Carcinoid tumors are rare thoracic neuroendocrine neoplasms that range from low-grade typical tumors to intermediate-grade atypical aggressive carcinoids and high-grade small cell carcinoma.[30] These tumors may secrete peptide hormones and neuroamines such as ACTH, serotonine, somatostatin, and bradikinin. Both sexes are affected in equal proportions, and patients are usually in their

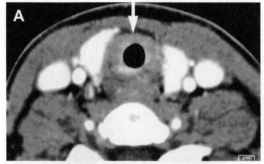

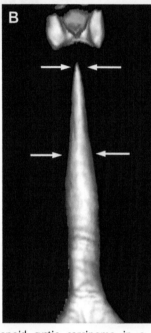

Fig. 3. Adenoid cystic carcinoma in a 50-year-old woman. (*A*) Axial CT after contrast media administration shows circumferential narrowing caused by circumferential wall thickening of the upper trachea (*arrow*). (*B*) Three-dimensional reconstruction of the trachea demonstrates the longitudinal extent of the tumor (*arrows*).

40s, whereas carcinoid is the most frequent bronchial tumor in childhood. No relation was found to cigarette smoking. Symptoms related to tracheobronchial obstruction and hemoptysis are by far more frequent than symptoms caused by ectopic secretion of hormones. In most cases (80%) these tumors are centrally located within the airways, affecting the main, lobar, and segmental bronchi. Tracheal involvement is exceptional. Carcinoid tumors classically appear as smooth, polypoid, cherry-red endobronchial masses at bronchoscopy. Although histologic diagnosis can be made with endoscopic biopsies, there is a high risk of hemoptysis.

Imaging presentation of centrally located carcinoids is similar for typical and atypical cases. In

most cases, carcinoids are endobronchial but also can be partially encased in the bronchial wall, creating an iceberg growth pattern, which is nicely demonstrated using CT and multiplanar reconstructions. In some cases (up to 60%), CT demonstrates marked homogeneous early contrast enhancement of an endobronchial nodule that reflects the rich vascularity of the carcinoid tumor (Fig. 5).[31] This pattern is highly suggestive of bronchial carcinoid tumor but is not always present. Differential diagnosis of endobronchial tumors with marked contrast enhancement on early phase dynamic contrast-enhanced CT detects even rarer neoplasms, such as glomus tumor[32] and hemangioma.[33] Intratumoral calcifications are reported in approximately 25% of cases (Fig. 6).[31] In some cases, bronchial carcinoid tumors produce complete obstruction of the bronchial lumen and subsequent atelectasis of the distal lung. In case of partial obstruction, expiratory air trapping can be demonstrated.

Hilar or mediastinal enlargement of lymph nodes can be present and is often related to inflammatory reaction from recurrent pulmonary infection. Lymph node metastasis of carcinoid tumor also may occur, more frequently in atypical carcinoid tumors.

OTHER PRIMARY MALIGNANT NEOPLASMS

Other malignant neoplasms are listed in Table 1. Their imaging presentation is not specific except for chondrosarcoma, which shows foci of calcifications within a mass.

LYMPHOMA

Primary malignant lymphoma of the trachea is rare. It is usually related to the mucosa-associated lymphoid tissue, a low-grade malignancy.[34] Clinical presentation is nonspecific. CT can reveal focal tracheal narrowing caused by a solitary mass (Fig. 7) or polypoid thickening of the tracheobronchial wall caused by diffuse infiltration of the submucosa.

SECONDARY TRACHEAL MALIGNANCY

Direct invasion of the central airways by neoplasms of the thyroid, esophagus, lung, and larynx is much more frequent than hematogenous metastases. In case of massive direct invasion, CT demonstrates the primary neoplasm and its extension by contiguity to the main airways. The signs associated with tracheal invasion are evidence of an endoluminal mass, the destruction of the cartilage, or a tracheoesophageal or bronchoesophageal fistula (Fig. 8).[35] Many cancers have the potential to metastasize to the trachea and

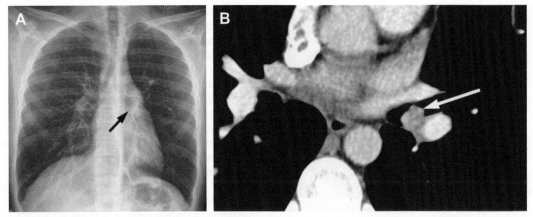

Fig. 4. Mucoiepidermoid carcinoma in a 23-year-old man who presented with hemoptysis. (*A*) Anteroposterior chest radiograph shows an endoluminal mass within the distal left mainstem bronchus (*arrow*). (*B*) Axial CT after contrast enhancement shows a 12-mm polypoid endobronchial mass slightly enhanced (*arrow*).

bronchi, such as breast, colorectal, renal, lung, ovarian, thyroid, uterine, and testicular and melanomas and sarcomas. The incidence of tracheal metastases in nonpulmonary malignancies is highly variable, ranging from 0.44% to 50%, according to their definition.[36] The overall incidence of tracheal metastasis in surgically resected non–small cell lung cancer was 0.44%; it was 0.77% in SCC and 0.18% in adenocarcinoma.[36] Endotracheal metastases of nonpulmonary cancers arise with a mean recurrence interval of 50.4 to 65.3 months[37] compared to a mean recurrence interval of 25.8 months in patients who present with lung malignancies. Endotracheal or endobronchial metastases appear as endotracheal nodules or

eccentric thickening of the airway wall (**Fig. 9**) or soft-tissue density with contrast enhancement. Histopathologic examination of tracheal biopsy specimens demonstrates the diagnostic of metastasis.

BENIGN TUMORS

Benign tumors of the central airways are rare and account for less than 2% of all lung neoplasms.[4] They can be of epithelial, mesenchymal, neural, or composite origin.[38] These tumors appear in clinical practice as the differential diagnosis of malignant lesions that are much more common. Although fiberoptic bronchoscopy

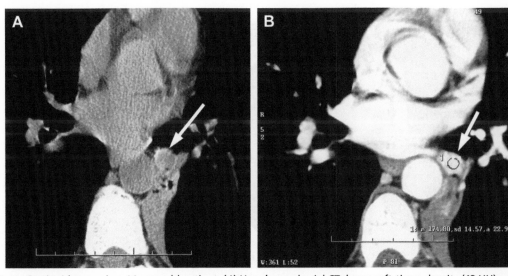

Fig. 5. Carcinoid tumor in a 14-year-old patient. (*A*) Unenhanced axial CT shows soft-tissue density (42 UH) nodule within the B6 bronchus and distal atelectasis (*arrow*). (*B*) Contrast-enhanced CT shows marked contrast enhancement of the nodule (174 UH) (*arrow*).

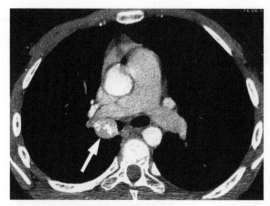

Fig. 6. Carcinoid tumor obstructing the right main stem bronchus. The tumor contains foci of calcifications and has an iceberg growth pattern (*arrow*).

identifieslesions within the airways, biopsies are often noncontributive because of severe inflammatory reaction in the periphery of the tumor. Chest radiography is usually unremarkable.[5] MDCT with thin collimation allows precise analysis of tissue attenuation of the lesions, enhancing in some cases the diagnostic capabilities of CT (**Box 1**). CT usually shows masses that are confined within the tracheobronchial lumen without evidence of invasion of surrounding structures.[39] Ko and colleagues[39] recently reported on a large series of 17 patients with pathologically proven benign tumors of the central airways.

HAMARTOMA

Hamartomas represent 3% to 10% of intrathoracic hamartomas.[40] These mesenchymal tumors are composed of a mixture of fat, cartilage, fibrous tissue, and an epithelial component. Endobronchial hamartomas arise more commonly in segmental bronchi;[41] tracheal location is unusual.[42] Radiologically, hamartomas are round, well-circumscribed lesions ranging from 0.5 to 3 cm in diameter. Demonstration of fat and calcifications within the lesion, which is considered diagnostic when present (**Fig. 10**),[43] is facilitated by using isotropic MDCT acquisitions with limited volume averaging effect. The fatty content or the calcifications may not be identified on CT, however,[42] and hamartoma appears as a nonspecific soft tissue mass. Goodman and colleagues[44] described a unique case of peripheral hamartoma arising from peripheral lung tissue with proximal extension and subsequent obstruction of the large airways. Because the tumor is slow growing, it may be responsible for bronchial obstruction and irreversible damage of the underlying lung. Hamartomas that develop within the airways require surgical treatment.

LIPOMA

Lipomas (0.1% of benign lung tumors) are often pedunculated and arise from the submucosal or interstitial adipose tissue of the central airways. Bronchial obstruction is frequent and responsible for atelectasis and postobstructive pneumonitis. As for other slow-growing endobronchial tumors, fiberoptic bronchoscopy is often nondiagnostic because of the fibrous capsule surrounding the lesions that may present with atypical inflammatory cells, leading to an incorrect diagnosis of

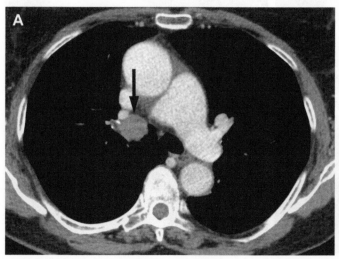
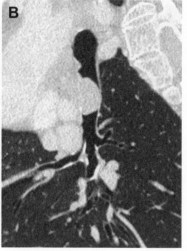

Fig. 7. Endobronchial mucosa-associated lymphoid tissue of the right main bronchus in an 80-year-old patient. (*A*) Axial CT after IV contrast media administration shows a 1.6-cm soft-tissue density mass (*arrow*). (*B*) Coronal oblique reformation of the tumor demonstrates the relationship with the bronchial tree.

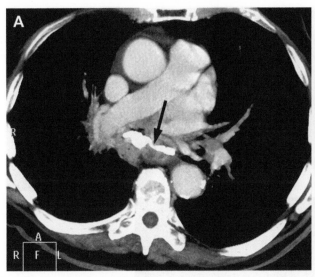

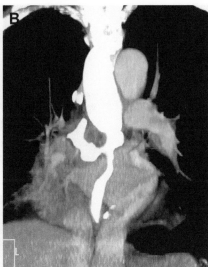

Fig. 8. Tracheoesophageal fistula in a patient with esophageal cancer extending to the right main bronchus. CT is acquired after contrast media opacification of the esophagus. (*A*) Axial CT shows the fistula between the esophagus and the right main bronchus (*arrow*). (*B*) Coronal maximum intensity projection provides a CT esophagogram, which shows the narrowed esophagus, the fistula, and the dilated esophagus above the cancer.

chronic inflammation or even bronchogenic carcinoma.[39] In those cases, CT is diagnostic when it shows the fatty density of the lesion without any calcification (**Fig. 11**).[45,46] A correct preoperative diagnosis may prevent lobectomy or pneumonectomy, because laser resection by means of

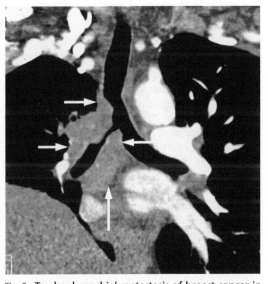

Fig. 9. Tracheobronchial metastasis of breast cancer in a 65-year-old woman. Coronal reformation shows soft-tissue density infiltration of the wall of the distal trachea extending to the right main bronchus (*arrows*), responsible for a severe narrowing of the right main bronchus lumen.

bronchoscopy is the treatment of choice for endoluminal lipomas.

GRANULAR CELL TUMORS (ABRIKOSSOFF'S TUMOR OR MYOBLASTOMA)

Granular cell tumors are uncommon benign neoplasms of neuroectodermal origin that are mainly located in the head and neck region.[2] They are discovered in the fourth decade of life and are more common in women. Pathologically, these tumors show a characteristic appearance; the cells are polymorphic and are embedded in various amounts of connective or reticular tissues. Mitoses are uncommon. The tumors are circumscribed but not encapsulated. At the level of central airways, they appear as polypoid masses of soft tissue density that may totally obstruct bronchi. Differentiation of granular cell tumors

---

Box 1
CT pathologic correlation in central airways neoplasms

Fat attenuation: lipoma, hamartochondroma

Calcification: hamartoma, chondroma, carcinoid

Fat and calcification: hamartoma

High contrast-enhanced tumor: carcinoid, hemangioma, glomus tumor, fibroma

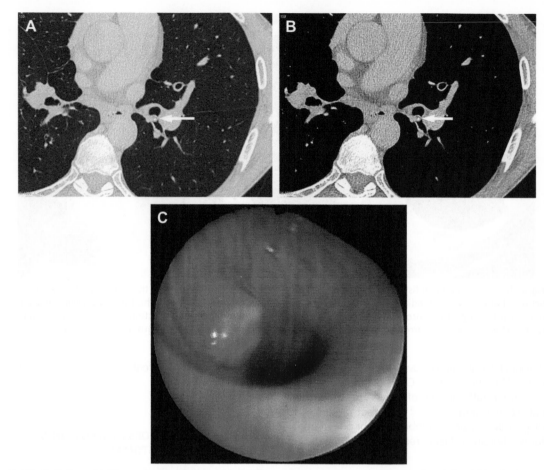

Fig. 10. Endobronchial hamartoma. (*A*) Axial CT without contrast shows an endoluminal nodule within the lumen of left B6 (*arrow*). (*B*) Axial CT (mediastinal window) shows fat and small calcifications within the lesion (*arrow*). (*C*) Bronchoscopy confirmed the diagnosis.

from carcinomas on the basis of imaging findings is not possible.

PAPILLOMAS

Inflammatory papillomas or polyps are associated with chronic irritation of the airways and occur with endobronchial foreign bodies, broncholithiasis, or exposure to gases. Squamous cell papilloma is one of the most common benign neoplasms of the central airways. It involves the larynx, bronchi, and infrequently the trachea, predominantly in middle-aged men with a history of smoking. The tumor appears as a lobulated, well-limited polypoid nodule within the airways without fatty content or calcification.[47]

Laryngotracheal papillomatosis is caused by infection with human papillomavirus. It can be contracted at birth or acquired through sexual transmission. The lesion arises in the larynx and spreads by seeding from the upper airways to the trachea in approximately 5% of cases.[48] Two third of patients are diagnosed before age 5. Papillomas are cauliflower lesions that enlarge around a central fibrovascular core on the central airway mucosal surface. These strictly endoluminal lesions appear on CT as single or multiple nodular irregularities of soft-tissue density, 0.5 to 1.5 mm in diameter in the tracheal or bronchial lumen (Fig. 12).[49] When extended to the lung parenchyma (< 1% of cases of laryngotracheal papillomatosis), papillomatosis produces nodules that may cavitate and form thin-walled cavities.[48] Lesions of papillomatosis are central and peripheral but with a predominance within the posterior half of the thorax. These lesions may transform into carcinoma and involve careful follow-up.

CHONDROMA

These rare benign cartilaginous tumors rarely develop in the trachea. CT may show foci of

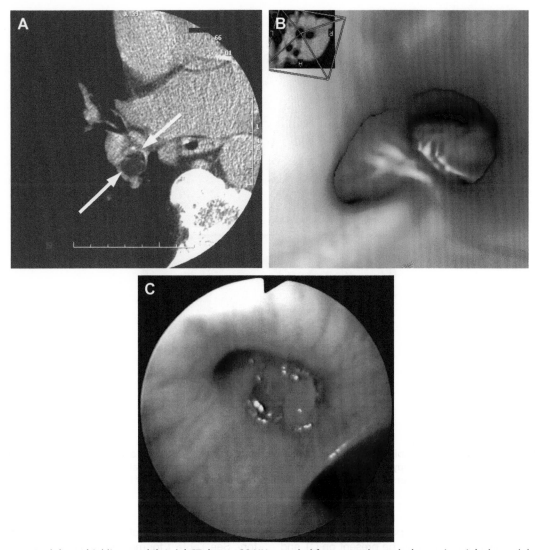

Fig. 11. Endobronchial lipoma. (*A*) Axial CT shows -90 HU rounded fatty mass (*arrow*) obstructing right lower lobe bronchus. VB (*B*) and real bronchoscopy (*C*) show excellent correlation.

calcifications within a sharply defined polypoid lesion up to 3 cm in diameter.[50] Imaging is unable to differentiate a chondroma from a chondrosarcoma; however.

SCHWANNOMA

This neurogenic tumor is rare and may present at any age. It is composed of Schwann's cells of nerve sheath. Most cases occur in adults. They are typically unique encapsulated tumors attached to a nerve but contain no axon protruding within the airways.[51] On CT, schwannoma appears as a well-limited mass of low tissue density before contrast administration; the mass is homogeneously and strongly enhanced after contrast

administration. Definitive diagnosis is demonstrated by biopsy under bronchoscopy.

ADENOMA

Pedonculated tracheobronchial adenoma (adenomatous polyp or mucous gland cystadenoma) arises from bronchial mucous glands and is rare. It appears as a solitary, spherical, soft-tissue density polypoid mass.[52]

LEIOMYOMA

This rare tumor accounts for approximately 2% of surgically resected benign lung tumors. Most leiomyomas are seen within the bronchi (70% of cases); 30% are detected in the trachea.[53]

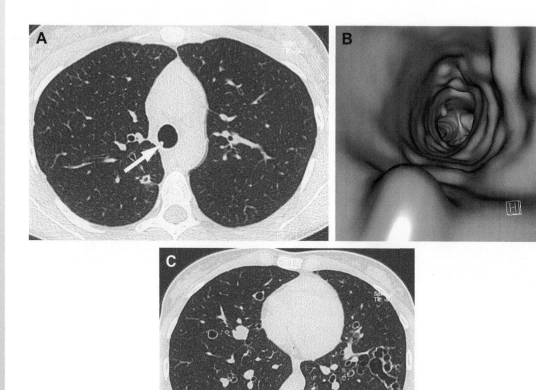

Fig. 12. Tracheobronchial papillomatosis in a 23-year-old man. (*A*) Axial CT shows a small, well-limited nodule (*arrow*). (*B*) Virtual endoscopy demonstrates multiple elevations of the tracheal wall caused by papillomas. (*C*) Axial CT at the level of lower lobes shows bilaterally distributed cysts. (*Courtesy of* D. Tack, MD, PhD, Baudour, Belgium.)

An iceberg tumor growth pattern with a large extraluminal component may be present on CT and should contraindicate bronchoscopic resection of these tumors. CT description of leiomyomas in the airways was reported by Kim and colleagues[53] in a series of 13 tumors: 2 were not depicted using CT because of their small size; 11 (84%) were identified using CT (9 as intraluminal nodules and 2 as iceberg tumors). Tumors are usually oval and are rarely lobulated or round. Obstructive pneumonia, atelectasis, or mucus plugging was present in 38% of cases. Calcifications are rare and are reported in less than 10% of cases. Most of these tumors appear as homogeneous nodules before contrast administration and become slightly enhanced after IV contrast injection.

OTHER BENIGN NEOPLASMS

Other neoplasms usually appear as smooth, polypoid, noncalcified nodules or masses limited to the airway wall. Histologic diagnosis is mandatory. See Table 1 for more examples.

DIFFERENTIAL DIAGNOSIS
Mucoid Pseudotumor

Mucus is the most commonly encountered soft-tissue mass within the airways, creating a mucoid pseudotumor. In most cases, mucoid pseudotumor is easily identified because the lesion is of low tissue attenuation, does not enhance after contrast media administration, may contain small air bubbles, is located in the dependant portions of the airway, is not associated with disruption of the cartilaginous rings of the trachea, and is mobile after coughing. In rare cases, thick mucus does not contain air, adheres to the wall of the airway, is not mobile after coughing, and may be mistaken for a real tumor (Fig. 13). Such false-positive CT findings are diagnosed using fiberoptic bronchoscopy.

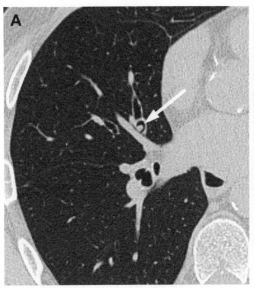 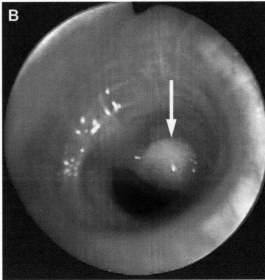

Fig. 13. Mucoid impaction mimicking endobronchial tumor. (*A*) Axial CT shows small, well-defined nodule within the right middle lobe bronchus (*arrow*). (*B*) Bronchoscopy demonstrates the mucous nature of the lesion (*arrow*).

Focal Infection

Focal infection may be responsible for tumor-like lesions when it produces granulation or endoluminal masses. Diagnosis is impossible with CT and requires fiberoptic bronchoscopy and microbacterial analysis. Specific pathogens include *Mycobacterium tuberculosis*, mucormycosis, *Klebsiella rhinoscleromatis*, and actinomycosis (**Fig. 14**).[54]

Broncholithiasis

Broncholithiasis may mimic a centrally located obstructive tumor on bronchoscopy. In these cases,

CT is more sensitive than bronchoscopy by identifying intraluminal and peribronchial calcifications distal to inflammatory airways stenosis.[55]

Tracheopathia Osteoplastica

Tracheopathia osteoplastica occurs almost exclusively in men over 50 years old; most patients are asymptomatic. This benign condition of unknown origin is characterized by multiple submucosal osteocartilaginous growths localized along the inner anterior and lateral walls of the trachea.[56] CT shows multiple irregular sessile nodules, 1 to 5 mm in diameter, that can be calcified protruding

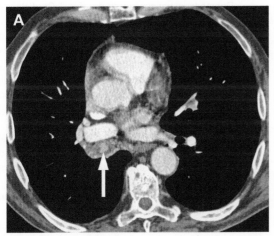 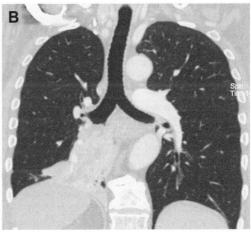

Fig. 14. Endobronchial actinomycosis mimicking endobronchial tumor. (*A*) Contrast-enhanced CT at the level of the right intermediate bronchus demonstrates complete occlusion of the bronchus (*arrow*). (*B*) Coronal reformation shows right lower lobe atelectasis. (*Courtesy of* D. Tack, MD, PhD, Baudour, Belgium.)

into the tracheal lumen. The posterior wall of the trachea is free of nodules.

Amyloidosis

Amyloidosis of the trachea is a rare condition that produces diffuse or focal irregular narrowing of the lower airways secondary to the deposits of extracellular amyloid within the submucosa. Deposits may be diffuse or multifocal with or without calcifications. Solitary amyloid pseudotumors are less common than diffuse disease.[57] CT shows concentric thickening of the tracheal wall that may extend up to the lobar bronchi with subsequent narrowing of the air column. Nodulation, plaques, and calcifications may be present.

REFERENCES

1. Grillo HC, Mathisen DJ. Primary tracheal tumors: treatment and results. Ann Thorac Surg 1990;49(1): 69–77.
2. McCarthy MJ, Rosado-de-Christenson ML. Tumors of the trachea. J Thorac Imaging 1995;10(3):180–98.
3. Regnard JF, Fourquier P, Levasseur P. Results and prognostic factors in resections of primary tracheal tumors: a multicenter retrospective study. The French Society of Cardiovascular Surgery. J Thorac Cardiovasc Surg 1996;111(4):808–13.
4. Macchiarini P. Primary tracheal tumours. Lancet Oncol 2006;7:83–91.
5. Kwong JS, Muller NL, Miller RR. Diseases of the trachea and main-stem bronchi: correlation of CT with pathologic findings. Radiographics 1992;12: 645–57.
6. Boiselle PM, Lee KS, Ernst A. Multidetector CT of the central airways. J Thorac Imaging 2005;20:186–95.
7. De Wever W, Vandecaveye V, Lanciotti S, et al. Multidetector CT-generated virtual bronchoscopy: an illustrated review of the potential clinical indications. Eur Respir J 2004;23(5):776–82.
8. Grenier PA, Beigelman-Aubry C, Fétita C, et al. New frontiers in CT imaging of airway disease. Eur Radiol 2002;12(5):1022–44.
9. Ferretti G, Bricault I, Coulomb M. Virtual tools for imaging the thorax. Eur Respir J 2001;18:1–12.
10. Ravenel JG, McAdams HP, Remy-Jardin M, et al. Multidimensional imaging of the thorax: practical applications. J Thorac Imaging 2001;16(4):269–81.
11. Luccichenti G, Cademartiri F, Pezzella FR, et al. 3D reconstruction techniques made easy: know-how and pictures. Eur Radiol 2005;15(10):2146–56.
12. Ferretti GR, Knoplioch J, Bricault I, et al. Central airway stenoses: preliminary results of spiral-CT-generated virtual bronchoscopy simulations in 29 patients. Eur Radiol 1997;7:854–9.

13. Remy-Jardin M, Remy J, Artaud D, et al. Tracheobronchial tree: assessment with volume rendering. Technical aspects. Radiology 1998;208(2):393–8.
14. Remy-Jardin M, Remy J, Artaud D, et al. Volume rendering of the tracheobronchial tree: clinical evaluation of bronchographic images. Radiology 1998; 208:761–70.
15. Burke AJ, Vining DJ, McGuirt WF Jr, et al. Evaluation of airway obstruction using virtual endoscopy. Laryngoscope 2000;110(1):23–9.
16. Finkelstein SE, Summers RM, Nguyen DM, et al. Virtual bronchoscopy for evaluation of malignant tumors of the thorax. J Thorac Cardiovasc Surg 2002;123(5):967–72.
17. Ferretti GR, Thony F, Bosson JL, et al. Benign abnormalities and carcinoid tumors of the central airways: diagnostic impact of CT bronchography. AJR Am J Roentgenol 2000;174:1307–13.
18. McAdams HP, Goodman PC, Kussin P. Virtual bronchoscopy for directing transbronchial needle aspiration of hilar and mediastinal lymph nodes: a pilot study. AJR Am J Roentgenol 1998;170:1361–4.
19. Boiselle PM, Reynolds KF, Ernst A. Multiplanar and three-dimensional imaging of the central airways with multidetector CT. AJR Am J Roentgenol 2002; 179:301–8.
20. Ferretti GR, Kocier M, Calaque O, et al. Follow-up after stent insertion in the tracheobronchial tree: role of helical computed tomography in comparison with fiberoptic bronchoscopy. Eur Radiol 2003;13:1172–8.
21. Honings J, van Dijck JA, Verhagen AF, et al. Incidence and treatment of tracheal cancer: a nationwide study in the Netherlands. Ann Surg Oncol 2007;14(2):968–76.
22. Freitag L, Ernst A, Unger M, et al. A proposed classification system of central airway stenosis. Eur Respir J 2007;30(1):7–12.
23. Licht PB, Friis S, Pettersson G. Tracheal cancer in Denmark: a nationwide study. Eur J Cardiothorac Surg 2001;19:339–45.
24. Kim TS, Lee KS, Han J, et al. Sialadenoid tumors of the respiratory tract: radiologic-pathologic correlation. AJR Am J Roentgenol 2001;177(5):1145–50.
25. Kwak SH, Lee KS, Chung MJ, et al. Adenoid cystic carcinoma of the airways: helical CT and histopathologic correlation. AJR Am J Roentgenol 2004;183(2): 277–81.
26. Campistron M, Rouquette I, Courbon F, et al. Adenoid cystic carcinoma of the lung: interest of 18FDG PET/CT in the management of an atypical presentation. Lung Cancer 2008;59(1):133–6.
27. Yousem SA, Hochholzer L. Mucoepidermoid tumors of the lung. Cancer 1987;60(6):1346–52.
28. Kim TS, Lee KS, Han J, et al. Mucoepidermoid carcinoma of the tracheobronchial tree: radiographic and CT findings in 12 patients. Radiology 1999;212(3): 643–8.

29. Ishizumi T, Tateishi U, Watanabe S, et al. Mucoepidermoid carcinoma of the lung: high-resolution CT and histopathologic findings in five cases. Lung Cancer 2008;60(1):125–31.

30. Jeung MY, Gasser B, Gangi A, et al. Bronchial carcinoid tumors of the thorax: spectrum of radiologic findings. Radiographics 2002;22(2):351–65.

31. Paillas W, Moro-Sibilot D, Lantuejoul S, et al. Bronchial carcinoid tumors: role of imaging for diagnosis and local staging. J Radiol 2004;85:1711–9.

32. Akata S, Yoshimura M, Park J, et al. Glomus tumor of the left main bronchus. Lung Cancer 2008;60(1):132–5.

33. Rose AS, Mathur PN. Endobronchial capillary hemangioma: case report and review of the literature. Respiration 2008;76:221–4.

34. Fidias P, Wright C, Harris NL, et al. Primary tracheal non-Hodgkin's lymphoma: a case report and review of the literature. Cancer 1996;77(11):2332–8.

35. Rapp-Bernhardt U, Welte T, Budinger M, et al. Comparison of three-dimensional virtual endoscopy with bronchoscopy in patients with oesophageal carcinoma infiltrating the tracheobronchial tree. Br J Radiol 1998;71:1271–8.

36. Chong S, Kim TS, Han J. Tracheal metastasis of lung cancer: CT findings in six patients. AJR Am J Roentgenol 2006;186(1):220–4.

37. Kiryu T, Hoshi H, Matsui E, et al. Endotracheal/endobronchial metastases: clinicopathologic study with special reference to developmental modes. Chest 2001;119(3):768–75.

38. Shah H, Garbe L, Nussbaum E, et al. Benign tumors of the tracheobronchial tree: endoscopic characteristics and role of laser resection. Chest 1995;107(6):1744–51.

39. Ko JM, Jung JI, Park SH, et al. Benign tumors of the tracheobronchial tree: CT-pathologic correlation. AJR Am J Roentgenol 2006;186:1304–13.

40. Arrigoni MG, Woolner LB, Bernatz PE, et al. Benign tumors of the lung: a ten-year surgical experience. J Thorac Cardiovasc Surg 1970;60(4):589–99.

41. Cosío BG, Villena V, Echave-Sustaeta J, et al. Endobronchial hamartoma. Chest 2002;122(1):202–5.

42. Reittner P, Müller NL. Tracheal hamartoma: CT findings in two patients. J Comput Assist Tomogr 1999;23(6):957–8.

43. Ahn JM, Im JG, Seo JW, et al. Endobronchial hamartoma: CT findings in three patients. AJR Am J Roentgenol 1994;163(1):49–50.

44. Goodman A, Falzon M, Gelder C, et al. Central airway obstruction caused by a peripheral hamartoma. Lung Cancer 2007;57(3):395–8.

45. Mata JM, Cáceres J, Ferrer J, et al. Endobronchial lipoma: CT diagnosis. J Comput Assist Tomogr 1991;15(5):750–1.

46. Raymond GS, Barrie JR. Endobronchial lipoma: helical CT diagnosis. AJR Am J Roentgenol 1999;173(6):1716.

47. Naka Y, Nakao K, Hamaji Y, et al. Solitary squamous cell papilloma of the trachea. Ann Thorac Surg 1993;55(1):189–93.

48. Kramer SS, Wehunt WD, Stocker JT, et al. Pulmonary manifestations of juvenile laryngotracheal papillomatosis. AJR Am J Roentgenol 1985;144(4):687–94.

49. Chang CH, Wang HC, Wu MT, et al. Virtual bronchoscopy for diagnosis of recurrent respiratory papillomatosis. J Formos Med Assoc 2006;105(6):508–11.

50. Frank JL, Schwartz BR, Price LM, et al. Benign cartilaginous tumors of the upper airway. J Surg Oncol 1991;48(1):69–74.

51. Righini CA, Lequeux T, Laverierre MH, et al. Primary tracheal schwannoma: one case report and a literature review. Eur Arch Otorhinolaryngol 2005;262(2):157–60.

52. Newhause MT, Martin L, Kay JM, et al. Laser resection of a pedunculated tracheal adenoma. Chest 2000;118:262–5.

53. Kim YK, Kim H, Lee KS, et al. Airway leiomyoma: imaging findings and histopathologic comparisons in 13 patients. AJR Am J Roentgenol 2007;189(2):393–9.

54. Naidich DP, Webb WR, Grenier PA, et al. Imaging of the airways: functional and radiologic correlations. Philadelphia: Lippincott Williams & Wilkins; 2005. 70–105.

55. Conces DJ, Tarver RD, Vix VA. Broncholithiasis: CT features in 15 patients. AJR Am J Roentgenol 1991;157:249–53.

56. Stark P. Radiology of the trachea. New York: Thieme Medical; 1991. p. 1–37.

57. Kirchner J, Jacobi V, Kardos P, et al. CT findings in extensive tracheobronchial amyloidosis. Eur Radiol 1998;8:352–4.

Nonneoplastic Tracheal and Bronchial Stenoses

Philippe A. Grenier, MD[a],*, Catherine Beigelman-Aubry, MD[a],
Pierre-Yves Brillet, MD, PhD[b]

KEYWORDS

- Tracheal stenosis • Bronchial stenosis
- Infectious tracheobronchitis • Relapsing polychondritis
- Wegener's granulomatosis • Tracheobronchial amyloidosis

Large airway diseases that may result in airway stenosis are neoplastic or nonneoplastic in origin. Tracheal and bronchial neoplasms are described in another article in this issue. Nonneoplastic diseases of central airways that may lead to airway lumen narrowing include iatrogenic strictures, infectious tracheobronchitis, systemic disease, saber sheath deformity of the trachea, tracheobronchopathia osteochrondroplastica, and broncholithiasis. Systemic diseases include amyloidosis, inflammatory bowel disease, relapsing polychondritis, sarcoidosis, and Wegener's granulomatosis. Tracheobronchomalacia that induces airway narrowing only during expiratory maneuver or cough is described in another article. Clinical recognition of tracheobronchial stenosis is notoriously difficult, especially early in its course. Clinical symptoms of airway obstruction are late and nonspecific. Earlier diagnosis is often possible with the advent of routine CT imaging.

Multidetector computed tomography (MDCT) is the imaging modality of choice for assessing such diseases.[1–4] It is important to be aware of the limitations of the axial plane for assessing airway stenosis. Subtle airway stenosis may be missed, and the craniocaudal extent of disease may be underestimated. By providing a continuous anatomic display of the airways, multiplanar reformations along and perpendicular to the central axis of the airways, and the three-dimensional reconstruction images help circumvent these limitations.[5–7] Such multiplanar and three-dimensional images

help surgeons and interventional pulmonologists to select adequate procedures and determine response to treatment. The use of MDCT with thin collimation (0.6–1.5 mm) over the entire chest during a single breath hold at full inspiration allows acquisition of volumetric high resolution data sets. Reconstruction of axial overlapped thin slices permits multiplanar reformations of high quality and helps detect and characterize airway wall thickening and calcifications. Generally, intravenous contrast is not required for assessing nonneoplastic airway stenoses; however, it is recommended in cases in which there is a high likelihood of diseases in the adjacent lymph nodes and for cases in which neoplastic airway disease may be suspected.[8] Additional acquisition during dynamic expiration using low dose may be helpful to detect coexisting tracheal or bronchomalacia.[3,9]

When assessing airway narrowing, it is important to carefully assess the location and extent along the airways of the stenosis and characterize the presence, distribution, and type of airway wall thickening. Considering these factors in combination with associated features in the mediastinum, hilum, and lung parenchyma and pertinent clinical and laboratory data should allow radiologists to provide a limited number of differential diagnoses.

IATROGENIC STENOSIS

The most common iatrogenic airway stenoses are tracheal strictures secondary to intubation or

[a] Hôpital Pitié-Salpêtrière, Assistance Publique-Hôpitaux de Paris (APHP), Université Pierre et Marie Curie, Service de Radiologie Polyvalente, Diagnostique et Interventionnelle, 47/83 boulevard de l'Hôpital, 75651 Paris cedex 13, Paris, France
[b] Hôpital Avicenne, Assistance Publique-Hôpitaux de Paris (APHP), Université Paris XIII, UPRES EA 2363, Service de Radiologie, 125, route de Stalingrad, 93009 Bobigny, France
* Corresponding author.
E-mail address: philippe.grenier@psl.aphp.fr (P. A. Grenier).

Radiol Clin N Am 47 (2009) 243–260
doi:10.1016/j.rcl.2008.11.011
0033-8389/08/$ – see front matter © 2009 Elsevier Inc. All rights reserved.

tracheostomy and bronchial anastomosis stenosis after lung transplantation. Strictures of the trachea are usually secondary to damage from a cuffed endotracheal or tracheostomy tube. The prevalence of stenoses after endotracheal tube placement has decreased substantially to 1% since the introduction of low pressure cuff endotracheal tubes.[10] Conversely, the prevalence of tracheal stenosis after longstanding tracheostomy tube placement remains high, with a rate of approximately 30%.[11] Infection, mechanical irritation, steroid administration, use of positive pressure ventilation, and prolonged intubation may increase the risk of stenosis occurrence.

The principal site of stenosis after intubation is the subglottic region at the level of the endotracheal balloon. Strictures are believed to occur when the cuff pressure is high enough to impede local blood circulation, with resultant ischemic necrosis of the mucosa. The most susceptible portions of the trachea are those in which the mucosa overlies the cartilaginous rings, which subsequently soften and become fragmented with the risk of tracheomalacia. This phase is subsequently followed by granulation formation and fibrosis. Postintubation stenosis is characterized by eccentric or concentric tracheal wall thickening and associated luminal narrowing. The craniocaudal length usually ranges from 1.5 to 2.5 cm.[12] Posttracheostomy stenosis occurs most commonly at the stoma site or less commonly at the site where the tip of the tube has impinged on the tracheal mucosa. It involves 1.5 to 2.5 cm of tracheal wall.[12,13]

Patients with mild iatrogenic stenosis may be initially asymptomatic. When present, symptoms are often delayed several weeks after extubation and include dyspnea on exertion, stridor, or wheezing. MDCT is the imaging modality of choice for detecting and characterizing tracheal stenoses. On axial images, CT demonstrates eccentric or concentric soft-tissue thickening with associated luminal narrowing. Multiplanar and reformations along the long axis of the trachea and volume rendering reconstruction help assess the location and extent of the stenosis (Fig. 1). On longitudinal images, the focal and circumferential luminal narrowing may produce a characteristic "hourglass" configuration (Fig. 2).[8] Less commonly, tracheal or bronchial stenosis may present as a thin membrane or granulation tissue protruding into the airway lumen (Fig. 3). Interventional bronchoscopic (eg, balloon dilatation, stenting, or laser therapy) or surgical procedures (eg, resection and anastomosis) may be used to treat symptomatic tracheal stenosis.

After lung transplantation, bronchial anastomotic stenosis may occur in 10% to 15% of cases.[14,15] Risk factors include infection, rejection, and immunosuppression. Affected patients typically present with failure of anticipated improvements in symptoms in the first months after transplantation and decline in pulmonary function, especially the FEV_1. Severe stenosis may result in progressive airflow obstruction that is difficult to clinically differentiate from other causes of airflow limitation that may occur after lung transplantation, particularly obliterative bronchiolitis.[16] The diagnosis is obtained at bronchoscopy and shows a focal cicatricial narrowing at the anastomotic site. MDCT with multiplanar reformations and volume rendering techniques provides information on the length of the stenosis and the patency of the distal airways, which is important in planning treatment. CT findings consist of focal narrowing at the bronchial anastomotic site.[16] Virtual bronchoscopy assesses the grade of the stenosis with a good correlation with pulmonary function tests.[15] CT is also used to assess the patency of the airways distal to high-grade stenosis not traversable by the endoscope and assess the response to treatment in the follow-up. Treatment consists of balloon dilatation followed by placement of a stent.

TUBERCULOSIS

Tracheobronchial stenosis caused by tuberculosis may occur in the setting of acute infection or as late as 30 years after infection.[14] Endobronchial tuberculosis has been reported in 10% to 37% of patients with pulmonary tuberculosis, and a variable degree of stenosis has been reported to occur in 90% of cases.[14] Isolated tracheal involvement is likely a rare manifestation. Tuberculosis typically involves the distal trachea and proximal bronchi. Spread along peribronchial lymphatic channels seems to play a more important role than direct airway spread by infected sputum. Evidence supporting this hypothesis is that in many patients in whom the central airways biopsy is positive for tuberculosis, main tuberculous lesions are confined to the submucosa, with the mucosa either remaining intact or having only shallow ulceration.[17] Another mechanism is local extension from adjacent mediastinal tuberculosis lymphadenitis. The presence of lymphadenopathy contiguous to the tuberculous lesions in the trachea or main bronchi suggests that local extension is a probable mechanism (Fig. 4).[18]

Tuberculosis indirectly involves the bronchial wall, and the disease undergoes several evolutional stages, including early formation of tubercles in the submucosal layer, ulceration and necrosis of the mucosal wall, and healing with a variable degree

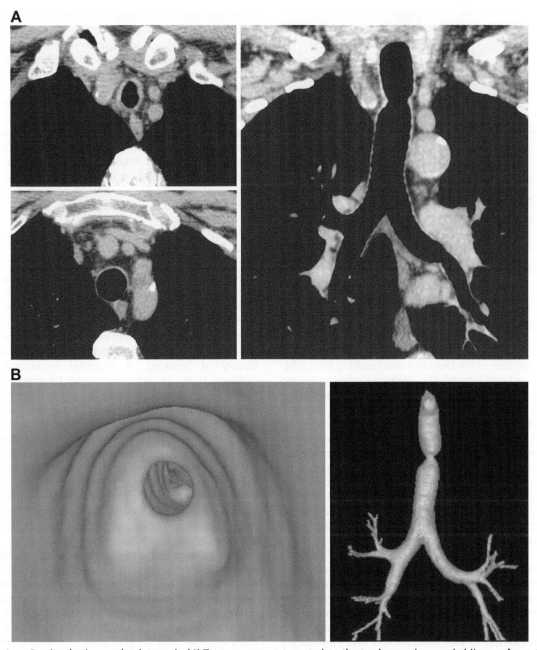

Fig. 1. Postintubation tracheal stenosis. (*A*) Transverse scans targeted on the trachea and coronal oblique reformat along the long axis and mainstem bronchi. (*B*) Descending virtual bronchoscopy and three-dimensional external rendering of the tracheobronchial tree. Presence of a short, concentric, and symmetric stenosis of the tracheal lumen at the level of the upper part of the intrathoracic portion of the trachea. Note on the transverse scan (*A*) a regular, concentric wall thickening at the level of the stenosis. Note calcifications of the aortic arch and right innominate artery.

of fibrosis or residual stenosis. Surprisingly, despite active infection, prebronchoscopic sputum samples produce negative results.[17] Endoscopic evaluation may not be diagnostic. Endobronchial biopsy has proven to be nonspecific in one third of the cases.[19] Although various stages of the disease may coexist in one patient, the prognosis is worse at the stage of fibrotic disease than in active disease. Not surprisingly, CT findings tend to reflect the stage of disease.[18–20] Stenosis in active disease occurs by hyperplastic changes and inflammatory edema. On CT scans, loss of

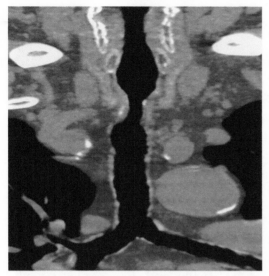

Fig. 2. Postintubation tracheal stenosis. Coronal obli-que reformation along the long axis of the trachea. Circumferential luminal narrowing extended along 2 cm associated with soft-tissue thickening, which produces the characteristic "hourglass configuration."

definition of the bronchial wall resulting from adjacent lymphadenopathy, irregular luminal narrowing with wall thickening, contrast enhancement of the tracheal wall, and rim enhancement of enlarged mediastinal node are common findings.[18–20] Rarely tuberculous nodes are observed to cavitate, which results in communication with the adjacent airway (see Fig. 4). Nodobronchial fistula is depicted by the presence of gas in cavitated hila or mediastinal lymphadenopathy adjacent to the airway. Discrete visualization of the sinus tract between the bronchial lumen and the hypertrophied cavitated lymph node can help plan therapy.

Stenosis in fibrotic disease occurs by fibrostenosis, and tuberculomas are usually absent in the diseased bronchial wall. On CT scans, smooth narrowing of the tracheobronchial lumen with minimal wall thickening is typically seen (Fig. 5). The bronchial stenosis is concentric with uniform thickening of the bronchial wall and involvement of the long segment of the bronchus (> 3 cm).[19] Unlike active infection, which involves the mainstem bronchi equally, fibrotic tuberculosis has been reported to involve the left mainstem bronchus more often.

CT findings of central airway tuberculosis are nonspecific and need to be distinguished from bronchogenic carcinoma affecting the central airways. The differential diagnosis from bronchogenic carcinoma can be made by the longer segment of involvement, circumferential luminal narrowing, and absence of an intraluminal mass. CT scans must always be supplemented by

bronchoscopy and biopsy to confirm the diagnosis, however. On follow-up after medical treatment, CT findings of irregular airway narrowing, obstruction, enlarged lymph nodes, and wall thickening, which are observed at the active stage of disease, are replaced by normal airways or smooth luminal narrowing with nearly normal wall thickness. In some patients, the airway disease progresses and residual fibrostenosis occurs. In fibrotic disease, usually there is no change in airway narrowing on follow-up CT studies. This disease form is resistant to medical treatment. Radiologic or surgical intervention is usually needed to restore the luminal patency.[14]

BRONCHIAL ANTHRACOFIBROSIS

Bronchial anthracofibrosis recently was defined as an inflammatory bronchial stenosis associated with anthracotic pigmentation on bronchoscopy without a relevant history of pneumoconiosis or smoking. Most patients with bronchial anthracosis have had no exposure to mining or industry and no history of smoking. A potential relationship between bronchial anthracosis and tuberculosis has been suggested, however. It has been hypothesized that the black pigments in the bronchial walls are derived from anthracotic material in the adjacent lymph nodes. The involved lymph nodes may perforate into the adjacent bronchi, and carbon particles in the lymph nodes may penetrate the bronchial wall as deep as the mucosa, resulting in coloring of the bronchial mucosa. Subsequently, healing with fibrotic response may occur and result in bronchial narrowing or obstruction with anthracotic pigmentation.[21,22]

Most patients are elderly women who usually present with cough, sputum, and dyspnea. On bronchoscopy, the right middle lobe bronchi is the most commonly involved site followed by the right upper, left upper, lingula division, right lower, and left lower lobe bronchi. Multiple site involvement may be seen in up to 50% of patients. On CT, a segmental collapse distal to the involved bronchi is the most commonly reported finding, with the right middle lobe being the most frequently involved lobe. The other findings include smooth bronchial narrowing accompanied by thickening of the wall and enlarged mediastinal or hilar lymph nodes adjacent to the involved bronchi (Fig. 6). Calcified nodes adjacent to the bronchi supplying the atelectatic lung are seen in more than 50% of patients. The CT findings are similar to those observed in bronchial tuberculosis. Bronchial biopsy is required to eliminate malignancy.

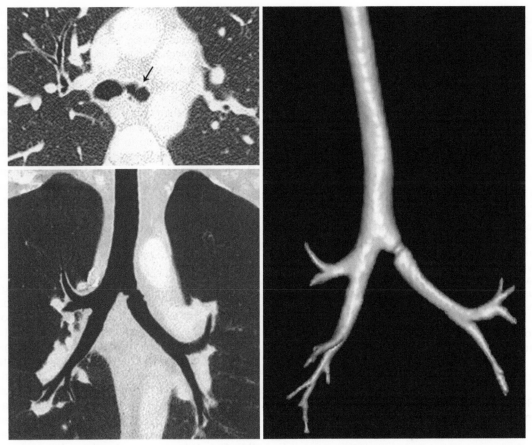

Fig. 3. Iatrogenic stenosis of the left mainstem bronchus occurred after a selective intubation. Transverse scan (*top left*), coronal oblique reformat of the tracheal lumen with minimum intensity projection (*bottom left*), and three-dimensional external rendering reformation of the tracheobronchial tree (*right*). The traumatic lesion occurred during intubation. Presence of nodular lesions along the inner surface of the left main bronchus (*arrow*) reflects granulation tissue and concentric narrowing of the origin of the left main bronchus.

RHINOSCLEROMA

Rhinoscleroma is a slowly progressive infectious granulomatous disease caused by *Klebsiella rhinoscleromatis,* a capsulated gram-negative bacterium that is endemic in tropical and subtropical areas.[23,24] Typically involving the upper respiratory tract, this organism also may involve the trachea and proximal bronchi. If left untreated, the infection progresses slowly over many years with alternating periods of remission and relapse. Pathologically in the granulomatous phase, nodules and masses cause partial obstruction of the involved airways (pseudoepitheliomatous hyperplasia). In the final sclerotic stage, the airway appears deformed, with stenosis developing secondary to fibrosis. The diagnosis is generally established by biopsy or positive culture results.

CT findings include diffuse nodular thickening of the proximal airway walls with luminal narrowing, nodularity of the tracheal mucosa, and concentric strictures of the trachea and bronchi. Mediastinal or hilar lymphadenopathy and postobstructive consolidation also may be present.[14] Antibiotherapy generally results in improvement, but advanced cases with fibrotic stenosis may benefit from interventional procedures.

FUNGAL TRACHEOBRONCHITIS

Acute tracheobronchitis caused by aspergillosis is uncommon and is usually restricted to the central airways. It usually occurs in severely immunocompromised individuals, especially persons with underlying malignancies or AIDS, or in individuals who have undergone bone marrow, lung, or heart transplantation.[25] Histologically, there is evidence of respiratory epithelial ulceration and submucosal inflammation. CT reveals nonspecific multifocal or diffuse tracheobronchial wall thickening, which results in either smooth or nodular luminal narrowing (**Fig. 7**).[26,27] Bronchial wall necrosis may lead

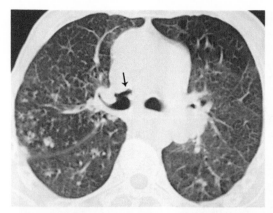

Fig. 4. Transverse scan in a patient with active tuberculosis. Nodobronchial fistula. There is direct communication between the anterior aspect of the right mainstem bronchus and the necrotic mediastinal lymphadenopathy (*arrow*). Multiple small, centrilobular, nodular opacities and nodules within the right upper lobe and, to a lesser extent, in the lower lobes represent endobronchial spread of tuberculosis.

to bronchial rupture, and associated rupture of the adjacent pulmonary artery may lead to death.[28]

RELAPSING POLYCHONDRITIS

Relapsing polychondritis is an unusual multisystemic disease of unknown origin that is

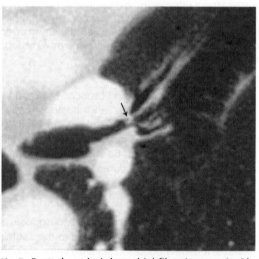

Fig. 5. Posttuberculosis bronchial fibrotic stenosis. Oblique reformat along the long axis of the left upper lobar bronchus. The bronchial stenosis visible at the origin of the lingular bronchus is short and has a nodular endoluminal appearance without any extrabronchial soft tissue mass (*arrow*). There is a distortion of the airways distal to the bronchial stenosis. (*From* Grenier PA. Imagerie thoracique de l'adulte. 3rd edition. Paris: Flammarion Médecine-Sciences; 2006; with permission.)

characterized by recurrent inflammation of the cartilaginous structures of the nose, external ear, peripheral joints, larynx, trachea, and bronchi.[29] Relapsing polychondritis is likely immune-mediated and considered to have an autoimmune pathogenesis. Although any age group may be affected, the peak of incidence of the disease is between the third and the sixth decades with a slight predominance in women. Airway involvement is present in up to 50% of patients and is a major cause of morbidity and mortality.[29,30] Rarely, it may occur as an isolated manifestation of the disease.[31] Airway involvement may be asymptomatic in early stages, but most patients with laryngotracheal involvement present with nonspecific respiratory tract symptoms, including cough, dyspnea, wheezing, aphonia, and hoarseness.[30]

The larynx and subglottic trachea are often the initial sites of involvement. As the disease progresses, the distal trachea and bronchi may be involved. The airway may be involved focally or diffusely. The distal bronchi may be involved to the level of the subsegmental bronchi. Pathologically, the disease is characterized by an acute inflammatory infiltrate in the cartilage and perichondrial tissue. Airway inflammation may result in luminal narrowing. Dissolution and fragmentation of the cartilage occur and may be followed by fibrosis.[32] In the late stages of the disease, this fibrosis-induced contraction of the airway may lead to severe luminal narrowing. Loss of structural cartilaginous support also may result in tracheobronchomalacia. The diagnosis of the disease is made on clinical criteria according to the lack of pathognomonic histologic or laboratory findings. Michet and colleagues[33] established major (auricular, nose, and laryngotracheal chondritis) and minor (ocular inflammation, hypoacousia, vestibular damage, seronegative inflammatory arthritis) criteria. The presence of two major criteria or one major criterion and two minor criteria permits the diagnosis.

The most common CT pattern is a combination of increased airway wall attenuation in association with smooth tracheal or bronchial wall thickening that characteristically spares the posterior membranous portion of the trachea (**Fig. 8**).[12–14,34] The degree of increased attenuation may range from subtle to a finding of frank calcification (see **Fig. 8A,B**).[34] Narrowing of airway lumen is more or less present (see **Fig. 8C**).[35] In advanced disease, circumferential wall thickening may be seen (**Fig. 9**). Gross destruction of the cartilaginous rings associated with fibrotic stenosis may occur. Important flaccidity of the airway wall may lead to

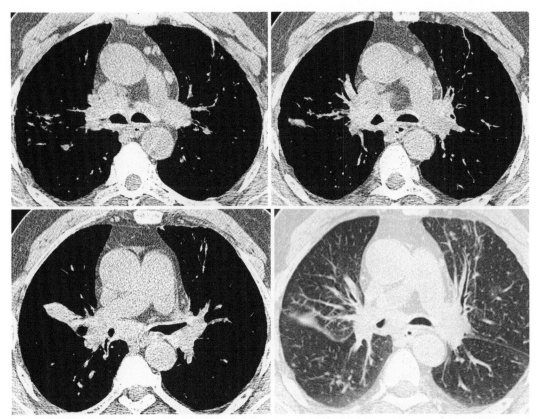

Fig. 6. Anthracofibrosis. Transverse nonenhanced CT scans. There is stenosis of the right upper lobar bronchus by a soft-tissue mass that extents medially into the mediastinum. Note thickening of the posterior wall of the right upper lobar and intermediate bronchi and narrowing and deformity of the lumen of the intermediate bronchus. Enlargement of the precarinal and subcarinal lymph nodes is visible.

considerable collapse on expiratory CT images (see **Fig.** 8D). Using dynamic expiratory CT, Lee and colleagues[9] found malacia and expiratory air trapping in 13 and 17 of 18 patients, respectively, with relapsing polychondritis.

Differential diagnosis is easy when CT images depict the presence of characteristic smooth thickening of the anterior and lateral walls of the trachea, and a diagnosis of relapsing polychondritis can be made with a high degree of confidence. Tracheobronchopathia osteoplastica, which also spares the posterior membranous wall of the trachea, is easily distinguished from relapsing polychondritis by the presence of nodules arising from the submucosa of the tracheal lumen and protruding into the airway lumen.

Treatment is based on a combination of medications, including corticosteroids, immunosuppressive agents, and nonsteroidal anti-inflammatory drugs.[29] Although these drugs may temporarily decrease the severity of recurrences, disease usually progresses. CT may play a role in the follow-up to assess the response to therapy.[36] Tracheostomy, tracheal stenting, and tracheal reconstruction may be used to provide long-term palliation.[37]

WEGENER'S GRANULOMATOSIS

Wegener's granulomatosis is a disease of unknown origin that is characterized by a necrotizing granulomatous vascularitis. Involvement of the large airways is a common manifestation of the disease. Its frequency was reported as 16% and 23% in two large series.[38,39] Although most often unassociated with symptoms or a late manifestation of well-established disease, tracheal or bronchial stenosis is occasionally responsible for the initial presentation.[40] Subglottic stenosis may occur in Wegener's granulomatosis without other evidence of pulmonary involvement. In one series, approximately 50% of tracheal stenoses occurred independently of other features of active Wegener's granulomatosis.[38]

Histologically, granulomatous inflammation and vascularitis typical of the disorder can be seen in the mucosa and submucosa in the early stage. Fibrosis is seen later. Endoscopic manifestations

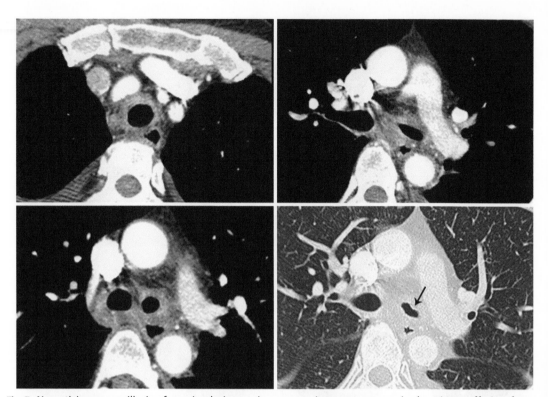

Fig. 7. Necrotizing aspergillosis of proximal airways in a young immunocompromised patient suffering from a B-lymphoma treated by chemotherapy and bone marrow transplantation. Transverse scans through the proximal airways. Diffuse and circumferential thickening of the tracheobronchial walls and soft tissue infiltration in the mediastinum fat around the trachea and mainstem bronchi are visible. There is regular narrowing of the left mainstem bronchus with a nodular appearance of the anterior inner surface of the left main bronchus (arrow).

include inflammatory tracheobronchial stenosis, ulcerating tracheobronchitis, and tracheobronchial stenosis without an inflammatory component. In a study of 77 patients with documented disease, Cordier and colleagues[41] found that 55% of patients in whom fiberoptic bronchoscopy was performed proved to have airway involvement. In another study by Daum and colleagues[42] that included 51 patients who underwent bronchoscopy, airway abnormalities were found in 59%, including subglottic stenosis in 17%, ulcerating tracheobronchitis in 60%, and tracheal or bronchial stenosis in 13%.

On CT, tracheal stenoses are most commonly subglottic (Fig. 10). In a study of ten patients with known tracheal involvement, Screaton and colleagues[43] noted that 90% of lesions were subglottic and identifiable as short segments of circumferential mucosal thickening. Usually tracheal stenosis presents as smooth or irregular circumferential narrowing approximately 2 to 4 cm long.[43,44] CT shows abnormal intratracheal soft tissue, which is often associated with thickening and calcification of the tracheal ring. Cartilaginous erosion also may be seen. CT studies

have demonstrated the high frequency of airway abnormalities on the more distal airways. For instance, Lee and colleagues[45] reported that central airway abnormalities could be identified in 30% of patients, whereas segmental and subsegmental bronchial wall thickening with or without luminal narrowing or obliteration was detectable in 73% of patients. Bronchial stenosis may result in distal collapse or consolidation of a lobe or lung.[41]

Virtual bronchoscopy may help detect subtle tracheal or bronchial stenosis. In a study of 18 virtual bronchoscopic examinations performed in 11 patients with Wegener's granulomatosis, 32 of 40 bronchoscopically visible stenoses, most in the lobar and intermediate bronchi, were identified on virtual bronchoscopy by at least one reading radiologist compared with only 22 on axial images.[46] According to the high prevalence of subglottic stenoses, this area always should be included in the imaging volume in patients with Wegener's granulomatosis.[8]

CT has proved valuable in follow-up of airway abnormalities. In the study by Lee and colleagues,[45] 20 patients had follow-up CT examinations. There was total resolution of previously

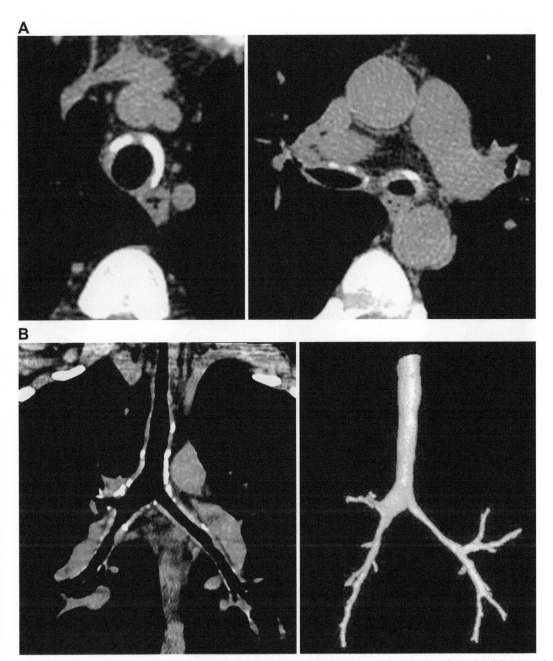

Fig. 8. Relapsing polychondritis. (*A*) Transverse scan through the trachea and mainstem bronchi. (*B*) Coronal oblique reformat along the proximal airways and three-dimensional external rendering of the tracheobronchial air content. (*C*) Transverse scan through the trachea and main and lobar bronchi. (*D*) Transverse scan of the carina at full inspiration (*top*) and during forced dynamic expiratory maneuver (*bottom*). There is diffuse and regular thickening of the anterior and lateral walls of the trachea and thickening of the anterior wall of the main and lobar bronchi. This wall thickening contains calcific deposits. Diffuse narrowing of the lumen of the mainstem and lobar bronchi is present. Tracheobronchomalacia with complete collapse of the mainstem bronchi during expiration was noted. (Fig. 8 *continued on next page*.)

C

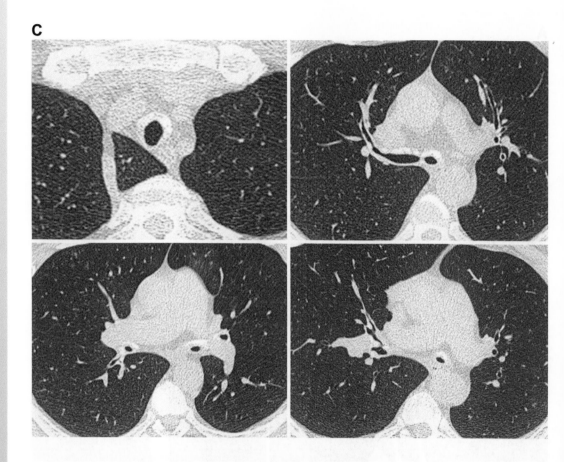

D

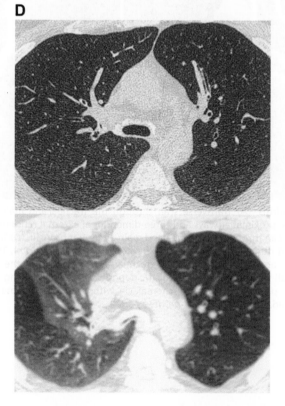

Fig. 8 (*continued*).

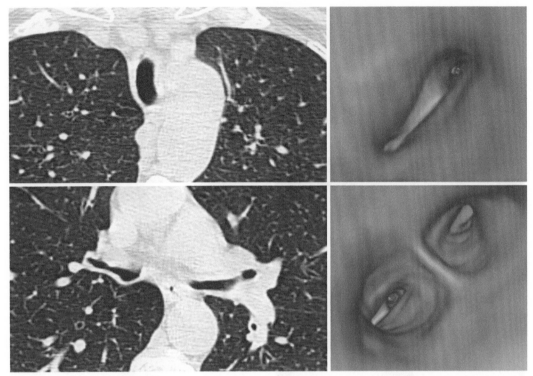

Fig. 9. Relapsing polychondritis in a patient with advanced disease. Transverse scan (*left*) and descending virtual endoscopic views (*right*). A circumferential wall thickening is present with narrowing and deformity of the tracheal and bronchial lumens.

identified airway abnormalities in 5 patients, lung parenchyma and airway lesions improved with partial disappearance in 12 patients, and 3 patients demonstrated evidence of recurrent disease. Tracheal stenosis is often unresponsive to systemic therapy, however, and local intervention is favored. Airway lesions may occur in the course of therapy, with symptomatic airway lesions occurring in the course of relapses.[47] CT may prove invaluable by demonstrating optimal sites for tracheostomy and by defining the true extent of disease when bronchial narrowing precludes complete bronchoscopic evaluation. Virtual bronchoscopy is particularly appreciated in this setting.[46] Park and colleagues[48] described MR findings of Wegener's granulomatosis stenosis. Abnormal soft tissue at the level of the stenosis is of intermediate signal on T1-weighted images, high signal on T2-weighted images, and enhances with contrast agent.

TRACHEOBRONCHIAL AMYLOIDOSIS

Deposition of amyloid in the tracheal bronchi may be seen in association with systemic amyloidosis or as an isolated manifestation.[49,50] Airway involvement may be focal, multifocal, or diffuse.

Diffuse involvement is most common. It may involve the larynx, trachea, main bronchi, and lobar or proximal segmental bronchi and often involves contiguous segments of the airway. Histologically the amyloid tends to be deposited initially in relation to tracheal gland acini and the walls of small blood vessels in the mucosa. As the amount of disease increases, the glands atrophy and the amyloid generates irregular plaques and nodules in the mucosa that are usually multifocal, or less commonly forms a single mass-like syndrome. The overlying mucosa is intact. Dystrophic calcification and ossification are frequently present at histologic examination.

Affected patients are often asymptomatic for a long time before diagnosis, which suggests that the disease progresses relatively slowly. In patients with proximal subglottic or laryngeal involvement, the disease manifests by hoarseness or stridor, whereas patients who have distal tracheal or bronchial involvement suffer from cough, wheezing, dyspnea, or hemoptysis.[49,50] In case of bronchial obstruction, patients may present with fever caused by obstructive pneumonitis. Endoscopic examination of the disease shows either submucosal plaques and nodules with a cobblestone appearance or a tumor-like

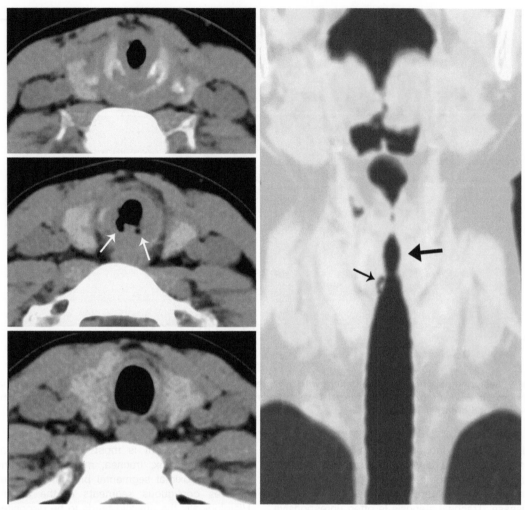

Fig. 10. Wegener's granulomatosis. Transverse scan over the upper part of the trachea (*left*) and coronal oblique reformat along the long axis of the trachea targeted on the larynx and cervical part of the trachea (*right*). Note short concentric stenosis of the subglottic area of the trachea (*large arrow*). Circumferential thickening of the tracheal wall at the level of the stenosis is visible. Note the presence of two small ulcerations within the posterior wall of the trachea (*small arrows*).

appearance or circumferential wall thickening. Endoscopic biopsies are diagnostic.[51]

On CT scans, amyloid results in circumferential tracheal or bronchial wall thickening caused by the submucosal deposition of nodules and plaques that induces a luminal narrowing (**Fig. 11**).[12,49,50,52–55] There may be multiple concentric or eccentric strictures. Mural calcifications are prominent features that have to be distinguished from calcified lymph nodes. Some patients with tracheobronchial amyloidosis have hilar or mediastinal calcified or noncalcified enlarged lymph nodes.[56] In patients with recurrent obstructive pneumonias, bronchiectasis also may be identified. Other patterns may be seen, such as eccentric strictures sparing the posterior

membrane of the trachea.[50] Local lesions give rise to endoluminal masses (amyloidomas) that may be radiologically indistinguishable from neoplasms.[8]

There have been rare reports of concurrent tracheobronchial amyloidosis and tracheobronchopathia osteoplastica.[49,51] In most cases, however, these entities prove pathologically distinct. In patients with severe narrowing, the amyloid deposits may be removed by intermittent bronchoscopic resections using either forceps or laser.[57] Resection is not curative, however, and lesions often recur 6 to 12 months after treatment. Other options include stenting and radiation therapy.[58,59] Tracheostomies may be required in case of subglottic involvement.

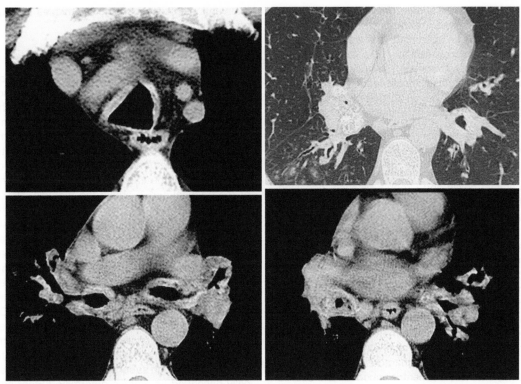

Fig. 11. Tracheobronchial amyloidosis as seen on transverse scans on the trachea and proximal bronchi. Thickening of the walls of the trachea is associated with tracheal lumen deformity. There is diffuse thickening of the bronchial walls containing calcific deposits. Luminal narrowing of the upper lobar and right intermediate bronchi and occlusion of the lumen of the right middle and lower lobar bronchi is visible.

SARCOIDOSIS

Involvement of the trachea is rare, and when it occurs, it is usually associated with laryngeal involvement.[60] The proximal and distal parts of the trachea may be affected, and the appearance of the stenosis may be smooth, irregular and nodular, or even mass-like. Bronchial involvement is much more common as a manifestation of sarcoidosis.[61] It was reported in 65% of 60 patients with sarcoidosis in a study by Lenique and colleagues[62] using high resolution computed tomography. The most common findings are regular or nodular bronchial wall thickening of the lobar, segmental, or subsegmental airways. The thickening likely reflects the presence of granulomas and fibrous tissue in the peribronchial interstitium. This bronchial wall thickening may result in smooth or irregular luminal narrowing, as was observed in 23% of patients by Lenique and colleagues (**Fig. 12**).[62] The luminal narrowing correlates with the presence of mucosal thickening at bronchoscopy and presumably reflects prominent inflammation in this location. Recognition of these abnormalities may be diagnostically important, because endobronchial biopsy of an abnormal site is likely to yield granulomas.

Obstruction of lobar or segmental bronchi may occur as a result of airway wall fibrosis and granulomas or peribronchial lymph node compression

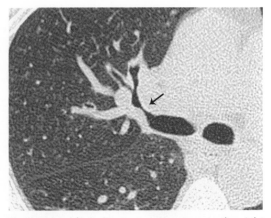

Fig. 12. Sarcoidosis. Transverse scan targets the right upper lobe. Stenosis of the distal part of the right upper lobar bronchus extending to the anterior segmental bronchus is visible (*arrow*).

and conglomerate fibrosis or some combination of these phenomena.[63] Lobar or segmental atelectasis remains an uncommon manifestation, occurring in approximately 1% of cases of sarcoidosis.[64] Bronchial stenosis caused by sarcoidosis may clear spontaneously or with steroid treatment.[65] Mechanical dilatation or stenting may be proposed in case of refractory stenosis.[66,67]

INFLAMMATORY BOWEL DISEASE

Chronic inflammatory bowel diseases, including ulcerative colitis and Crohn's disease, occasionally may demonstrate extraintestinal manifestations. Among them, airway disease is relatively uncommon and may take several forms, including ulcerative tracheitis and tracheobronchitis, bronchiectasis, and small airway disease, most commonly obliterative bronchiolitis.[68–70] Tracheobronchial complications are rare and occur more often in association with ulcerative colitis than Crohn's disease. In most—but not all—cases, the diagnosis of inflammatory bowel disease precedes the presence of airway disease.

Tracheobronchitis is characterized histologically by more or less concentric mucosal and submucosal fibrosis and chronic inflammation. Ulceration and luminal narrowing may be evident. The cartilaginous plates may be calcified but are not destroyed. Affected patients present with nonspecific symptoms of airway obstruction, including stridor, dyspnea, and cough. CT findings are nonspecific.[14] The tracheobronchial walls are thickened and produce irregular luminal narrowing. Bronchial wall thickening and bronchiectasis also may be present with or without mucoid impaction. If medical therapy (intravenous steroids and cyclosporine) fails to resolve symptoms, interventional bronchoscopic techniques may be considered.[8]

SABER SHEATH TRACHEA

Sabear sheath trachea is a relatively uncommon deformity of the trachea characterized by reduction in coronal diameter and elongation of the sagittal diameter. It is defined by a coronal diameter equal to or less than one-half its sagittal diameter, measured at 1 cm above the top of the aortic arch.[71,72] This deformity affects only the intrathoracic portion of the trachea, with abrupt widening of the tracheal lumen above the thoracic inlet. It may extend downward on the mainstem bronchi. This deformity is almost always associated with chronic obstructive pulmonary disease and has been described exclusively in men.[71] It has been postulated to be the consequence of abnormal pattern and magnitude pressure changes related to hyperinflated lungs.[13] The deformity is often detected incidentally on chest radiograph or CT (Fig. 13). The inner contour of the trachea is often smooth but occasionally has a nodular contour. Calcification of tracheal cartilage is frequently evident.[73] Although saber sheath trachea is classically described as a static deformity, further narrowing of the tracheal lumen can be documented when patients are examined during forced expiration, reflecting excessive collapsibility of lateral walls (tracheomalacia).[74]

TRACHEOBRONCHOPATHIA OSTEOCHONDROPLASTICA

This rare disorder is characterized by the presence of multiple submucosal cartilaginous or bony nodules projecting into the tracheobronchial lumen.[12–14,75] It is a benign disease of

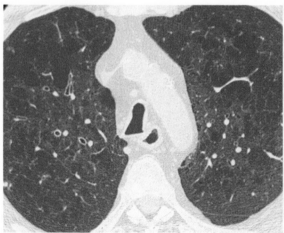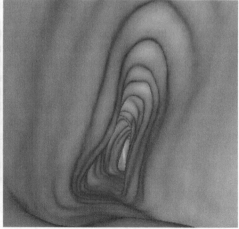

Fig.13. Saber sheath trachea in a patient with severe chronic obstructive pulmonary disease. Transverse scan (*left*) and descending virtual endoscopy view (*right*). Characteristic deformity of the tracheal lumen is present.

unknown origin. Men are more frequently involved than women, and most patients are older than age 50. Several potential causes or associations have been postulated, including amyloidosis, hereditary factors, chemical irritation, and infection. Most cases are asymptomatic, but patients may present with chronic cough, hoarseness, stridor, or wheezing that is sometimes confused with asthma. It has been reported to cause hemoptysis.[76] Histologically, the nodules are recognized as submucosal osteocartilaginous growths. The mucosal surface is intact, and a connection between the nodule and the perichondrium of the tracheal cartilaginous ring is frequently identified. Because it contains no cartilage, the posterior wall of the trachea is spared.

CT is the imaging modality of choice for this condition.[75,77–79] It demonstrates a pattern of multiple calcified nodules arising from the anterior and lateral walls of the trachea and protruding into the lumen. The nodules typically range in size from 3 to 8 mm. They result in diffuse luminal narrowing and are associated with thickening and deformity of the tracheal rings. The posterior membranous portion of the trachea is spared. The differential diagnoses include amyloidosis and tuberculosis, but these diseases do not respect the posterior wall. Relapsing polychondritis also affects the posterior wall, but the thickening of the wall is not nodular in appearance. In most patients, the disease progresses slowly. Therapy is requisite only when the tracheal or bronchial lumens become compromised. Therapeutic options include surgical or laser resection, radiation therapy, and stent placement.

BRONCHOLITHIASIS

Broncholithiasis is a condition in which calcified lymph nodes distort and erode into the tracheobronchial tree, and patients may expectorate or aspirate the calcified material.[80] Most broncholiths are composed of fragments of calcified material that were originally located in a peribronchial lymph node. Broncholithiasis is considered as a late complication of granulomatous lymphadenitis caused by *Mycobacterium tuberculosis* or fungi such as *Histoplasma capsulatum*. Pathologically the airway is fibrotic and distorted, and erosion by calcified lymph nodes may be apparent. Bronchial wall fibrosis and obstruction pneumonitis may be present. Identification of calcified material within an acute inflammatory exudate or granulation tissue is key for diagnosis on bronchoscopic biopsy specimen. The diagnosis may be made at CT by identifying a focus of calcified material within the bronchial lumen without any mass (**Fig. 14**).[80–82] Peribronchial

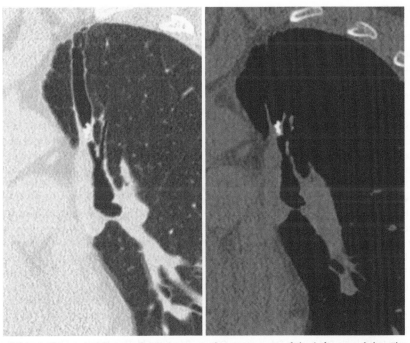

Fig.14. Broncholithiasis. Coronal oblique reformat targets the upper part of the left upper lobe. There is complete obliteration of the lumen of the subsegmental bronchus by endoluminal calcified material, complicated by post-obstructive bronchiectasis.

lymph node calcification is commonly seen. Post-obstructive abnormalities are often present, including bronchiectasis, obstructive consolidation, and air trapping.

SUMMARY

MDCT using thin collimation and postprocessing techniques, such as multiplanar reformations along and perpendicular to the central axes of the central airways, and volume rendering techniques, such as virtual bronchoscopy and virtual bronchography, has become the imaging modality of choice for the diagnosis of nonneoplastic tracheal and bronchial stenoses. It may ensure accurate assessment of the location and extent of the stenosis and good characterization of the presence, distribution, type, and calcification of airway wall thickening. The consideration of these abnormalities in combination with associated CT findings observed in the mediastinum, hilum, or lung parenchyma and available clinical and laboratory data help the radiologist to shorten the list of different diagnoses. The role of MDCT is also to guide surgical and interventional endoscopic procedures and assess response to treatment.

REFERENCES

1. Boiselle PM, Ernst A. Recent advances in central airway imaging. Chest 2002;121(5):1651–60.
2. Boiselle PM, Reynolds KF, Ernst A. Multiplanar and three-dimensional imaging of the central airways with multidetector CT. AJR Am J Roentgenol 2002; 179(2):301–8.
3. Grenier PA, Beigelman-Aubry C, Fetita C, et al. New frontiers in CT imaging of airway disease. Eur Radiol 2002;12(5):1022–44.
4. Salvolini L, Bichi Secchi E, Costarelli L, et al. Clinical applications of 2D and 3D CT imaging of the airways: a review. Eur J Radiol 2000;34(1):9–25.
5. Naidich DP, Gruden JF, McGuinness G, et al. Volumetric (helical/spiral) CT (VCT) of the airways. J Thorac Imaging 1997;12(1):11–28.
6. Remy-Jardin M, Remy J, Artaud D, et al. Volume rendering of the tracheobronchial tree: clinical evaluation of bronchographic images. Radiology 1998; 208(3):761–70.
7. Remy-Jardin M, Remy J, Artaud D, et al. Tracheobronchial tree: assessment with volume rendering: technical aspects. Radiology 1998;208(2):393–8.
8. Boiselle PM, Castena J, Ernst A, et al. Tracheobronchial stenosis. In: Boiselle PM, Lynch DA, editors. CT of the airways. Totowa (NJ): Humana Press; 2008. p. 121–49.
9. Lee KS, Ernst A, Trentham DE, et al. Relapsing polychondritis: prevalence of expiratory CT airway abnormalities. Radiology 2006;240(2):565–73.
10. Stauffer JL, Olson DE, Petty TL. Complications and consequences of endotracheal intubation and tracheotomy: a prospective study of 150 critically ill adult patients. Am J Med 1981;70(1):65–76.
11. Norwood S, Vallina VL, Short K, et al. Incidence of tracheal stenosis and other late complications after percutaneous tracheostomy. Ann Surg 2000; 232(2):233–41.
12. Webb EM, Elicker BM, Webb WR. Using CT to diagnose nonneoplastic tracheal abnormalities: appearance of the tracheal wall. AJR Am J Roentgenol 2000;174(5):1315–21.
13. Marom EM, Goodman PC, McAdams HP. Focal abnormalities of the trachea and main bronchi. AJR Am J Roentgenol 2001;176(3):707–11.
14. Prince JS, Duhamel DR, Levin DL, et al. Nonneoplastic lesions of the tracheobronchial wall: radiologic findings with bronchoscopic correlation. Radiographics 2002;22:S215–30.
15. Shitrit D, Valdsislav P, Grubstein A, et al. Accuracy of virtual bronchoscopy for grading tracheobronchial stenosis: correlation with pulmonary function test and fiberoptic bronchoscopy. Chest 2005;128(5): 3545–50.
16. McAdams HP, Palmer SM, Erasmus JJ, et al. Bronchial anastomotic complications in lung transplant recipients: virtual bronchoscopy for noninvasive assessment. Radiology 1998;209(3):689–95.
17. Lee JH, Park SS, Lee DH, et al. Endobronchial tuberculosis: clinical and bronchoscopic features in 121 cases. Chest 1992;102(4):990–4.
18. Kim Y, Lee KS, Yoon JH, et al. Tuberculosis of the trachea and main bronchi: CT findings in 17 patients. AJR Am J Roentgenol 1997;168(4):1051–6.
19. Choe KO, Jeong HJ, Sohn HY. Tuberculous bronchial stenosis: CT findings in 28 cases. AJR Am J Roentgenol 1990;155(5):971–6.
20. Moon WK, Im JG, Yeon KM, et al. Tuberculosis of the central airways: CT findings of active and fibrotic disease. AJR Am J Roentgenol 1997; 169(3):649–53.
21. Chung MP, Lee KS, Han J, et al. Bronchial stenosis due to anthracofibrosis. Chest 1998; 113(2):344–50.
22. Kim HY, Im JG, Goo JM, et al. Bronchial anthracofibrosis (inflammatory bronchial stenosis with anthracotic pigmentation): CT findings. AJR Am J Roentgenol 2000;174(2):523–7.
23. Amoils CP, Shindo ML. Laryngotracheal manifestations of rhinoscleroma. Ann Otol Rhinol Laryngol 1996;105(5):336–40.
24. Yigla M, Ben-Izhak O, Oren I, et al. Laryngotracheobronchial involvement in a patient with nonendemic rhinoscleroma. Chest 2000;117(6):1795–8.

25. Miller WT Jr, Sais GJ, Frank I, et al. Pulmonary aspergillosis in patients with AIDS: clinical and radiographic correlations. Chest 1994;105(1):37–44.

26. Franquet T, Muller NL, Oikonomou A, et al. Aspergillus infection of the airways: computed tomography and pathologic findings. J Comput Assist Tomogr 2004;28(1):10–6.

27. Franquet T, Serrano F, Gimenez A, et al. Necrotizing aspergillosis of large airways: CT findings in eight patients. J Comput Assist Tomogr 2002;26(3):342–5.

28. Taouli B, Cadi M, Leblond V, et al. Invasive aspergillosis of the mediastinum and left hilum: CT features. AJR Am J Roentgenol 2004;183(5):1224–6.

29. Trentham DE, Le CH. Relapsing polychondritis. Ann Intern Med 1998;129(2):114–22.

30. Letko E, Zafirakis P, Baltatzis S, et al. Relapsing polychondritis: a clinical review. Semin Arthritis Rheum 2002;31(6):384–95.

31. Tsunezuka Y, Sato H, Shimizu H. Tracheobronchial involvement in relapsing polychondritis. Respiration 2000;67(3):320–2.

32. Tillie-Leblond I, Wallaert B, Leblond D, et al. Respiratory involvement in relapsing polychondritis: clinical, functional, endoscopic, and radiographic evaluations. Medicine (Baltimore) 1998;77(3):168–76.

33. Michet CJ Jr, McKenna CH, Luthra HS, et al. Relapsing polychondritis: survival and predictive role of early disease manifestations. Ann Intern Med 1986;104(1):74–8.

34. Behar JV, Choi YW, Hartman TA, et al. Relapsing polychondritis affecting the lower respiratory tract. AJR Am J Roentgenol 2002;178(1):173–7.

35. Kilman WJ. Narrowing of the airway in relapsing polychondritis. Radiology 1978;126(2):373–6.

36. Im JG, Chung JW, Han SK, et al. CT manifestations of tracheobronchial involvement in relapsing polychondritis. J Comput Assist Tomogr 1988;12(5):792–3.

37. Sarodia BD, Dasgupta A, Mehta AC. Management of airway manifestations of relapsing polychondritis: case reports and review of literature. Chest 1999;116(6):1669–75.

38. Langford CA, Sneller MC, Hallahan CW, et al. Clinical features and therapeutic management of subglottic stenosis in patients with Wegener's granulomatosis. Arthritis Rheum 1996;39(10):1754–60.

39. McDonald TJ, Neel HB 3rd, DeRemee RA. Wegener's granulomatosis of the subglottis and the upper portion of the trachea. Ann Otol Rhinol Laryngol 1982;91(6 Pt 1):588–92.

40. Stein MG, Gamsu G, Webb WR, et al. Computed tomography of diffuse tracheal stenosis in Wegener granulomatosis. J Comput Assist Tomogr 1986;10(5):868–70.

41. Cordier JF, Valeyre D, Guillevin L, et al. Pulmonary Wegener's granulomatosis: a clinical and imaging study of 77 cases. Chest 1990;97(4):906–12.

42. Daum TE, Specks U, Colby TV, et al. Tracheobronchial involvement in Wegener's granulomatosis. Am J Respir Crit Care Med 1995;151(2 Pt 1):522–6.

43. Screaton NJ, Sivasothy P, Flower CD, et al. Tracheal involvement in Wegener's granulomatosis: evaluation using spiral CT. Clin Radiol 1998;53(11):809–15.

44. Cohen MI, Gore RM, August CZ, et al. Tracheal and bronchial stenosis associated with mediastinal adenopathy in Wegener granulomatosis: CT findings. J Comput Assist Tomogr 1984;8(2):327–9.

45. Lee KS, Kim TS, Fujimoto K, et al. Thoracic manifestation of Wegener's granulomatosis: CT findings in 30 patients. Eur Radiol 2003;13(1):43–51.

46. Summers RM, Aggarwal NR, Sneller MC, et al. CT virtual bronchoscopy of the central airways in patients with Wegener's granulomatosis. Chest 2002;121(1):242–50.

47. Aberle DR, Gamsu G, Lynch D. Thoracic manifestations of Wegener's granulomatosis: diagnosis and course. Radiology 1990;174(3 Pt 1):703–9.

48. Park KJ, Bergin CJ, Harrell J. MR findings of tracheal involvement in Wegener's granulomatosis. AJR Am J Roentgenol 1998;171(2):524–5.

49. Georgiades CS, Neyman EG, Barish MA, et al. Amyloidosis: review and CT manifestations. Radiographics 2004;24(2):405–16.

50. Kim HY, Im JG, Song KS, et al. Localized amyloidosis of the respiratory system: CT features. J Comput Assist Tomogr 1999;23(4):627–31.

51. Piazza C, Cavaliere S, Foccoli P, et al. Endoscopic management of laryngo-tracheobronchial amyloidosis: a series of 32 patients. Eur Arch Otorhinolaryngol 2003;260(7):349–54.

52. Kirchner J, Jacobi V, Kardos P, et al. CT findings in extensive tracheobronchial amyloidosis. Eur Radiol 1998;8(3):352–4.

53. Ozer C, Nass Duce M, Yildiz A, et al. Primary diffuse tracheobronchial amyloidosis: case report. Eur J Radiol 2002;44(1):37–9.

54. Pickford HA, Swensen SJ, Utz JP. Thoracic cross-sectional imaging of amyloidosis. AJR Am J Roentgenol 1997;168(2):351–5.

55. Urban BA, Fishman EK, Goldman SM, et al. CT evaluation of amyloidosis: spectrum of disease. Radiographics 1993;13(6):1295–308.

56. Crestani B, Monnier A, Kambouchner M, et al. Tracheobronchial amyloidosis with hilar lymphadenopathy associated with a serum monoclonal immunoglobulin. Eur Respir J 1993;6(10):1569–71.

57. Flemming AF, Fairfax AJ, Arnold AG, et al. Treatment of endobronchial amyloidosis by intermittent bronchoscopic resection. Br J Dis Chest 1980;74(2):183–8.

58. Kalra S, Utz JP, Edell ES, et al. External-beam radiation therapy in the treatment of diffuse

tracheobronchial amyloidosis. Mayo Clin Proc 2001;76(8):853–6.

59. Yang S, Chia SY, Chuah KL, et al. Tracheobronchial amyloidosis treated with rigid bronchoscopy and stenting. Surg Endosc 2003;17(4):658–9.

60. Brandstetter RD, Messina MS, Sprince NL, et al. Tracheal stenosis due to sarcoidosis. Chest 1981; 80(5):656.

61. Miller A, Brown LK, Teirstein AS. Stenosis of main bronchi mimicking fixed upper airway obstruction in sarcoidosis. Chest 1985;88(2):244–8.

62. Lenique F, Brauner MW, Grenier P, et al. CT assessment of bronchi in sarcoidosis: endoscopic and pathologic correlations. Radiology 1995;194(2): 419–23.

63. Olsson T, Bjornstad-Pettersen H, Stjernberg NL. Bronchostenosis due to sarcoidosis: a cause of atelectasis and airway obstruction simulating pulmonary neoplasm and chronic obstructive pulmonary disease. Chest 1979;75(6):663–6.

64. Freundlich IM, Libshitz HI, Glassman LM, et al. Sarcoidosis: typical and atypical thoracic manifestations and complications. Clin Radiol 1970;21(4):376–83.

65. Corsello BF, Lohaus GH, Funahashi A. Endobronchial mass lesion due to sarcoidosis: complete resolution with corticosteroids. Thorax 1983;38(2): 157–8.

66. Fouty BW, Pomeranz M, Thigpen TP, et al. Dilatation of bronchial stenoses due to sarcoidosis using a flexible fiberoptic bronchoscope. Chest 1994;106(3): 677–80.

67. Mayse ML, Greenheck J, Friedman M, et al. Successful bronchoscopic balloon dilation of nonmalignant tracheobronchial obstruction without fluoroscopy. Chest 2004;126(2):634–7.

68. Camus P, Colby TV. The lung in inflammatory bowel disease. Eur Respir J 2000;15(1):5–10.

69. Ulrich R, Goldberg R, Line WS. Crohn's disease: a rare cause of upper airway obstruction. J Emerg Med 2000;19(4):331–2.

70. Wilcox P, Miller R, Miller G, et al. Airway involvement in ulcerative colitis. Chest 1987;92(1):18–22.

71. Greene R. "Saber-sheath" trachea: relation to chronic obstructive pulmonary disease. AJR Am J Roentgenol 1978;130(3):441–5.

72. Trigaux JP, Hermes G, Dubois P, et al. CT of saber-sheath trachea: correlation with clinical, chest radiographic and functional findings. Acta Radiol 1994; 35(3):247–50.

73. Rubenstein J, Weisbrod G, Steinhardt MI. Atypical appearances of "saber-sheath" trachea. Radiology 1978;127(1):41–2.

74. Gamsu G, Webb WR. Computed tomography of the trachea: normal and abnormal. AJR Am J Roentgenol 1982;139(2):321–6.

75. Restrepo S, Pandit M, Villamil MA, et al. Tracheobronchopathia osteochondroplastica: helical CT findings in 4 cases. J Thorac Imaging 2004;19(2):112–6.

76. Briones-Gomez A. Tracheopathie osteoplastica. J Bronchol 2000;7:301–5.

77. Bottles K, Nyberg DA, Clark M, et al. CT diagnosis of tracheobronchopathia osteochondroplastica. J Comput Assist Tomogr 1983;7(2):324–7.

78. Mariotta S, Pallone G, Pedicelli G, et al. Spiral CT and endoscopic findings in a case of tracheobronchopathia osteochondroplastica. J Comput Assist Tomogr 1997; 21(3):418–20.

79. Onitsuka H, Hirose N, Watanabe K, et al. Computed tomography of tracheopathia osteoplastica. AJR Am J Roentgenol 1983;140(2):268–70.

80. Conces DJ, Tarver RD, Vix VA. Broncholithiasis: CT features in 15 patients. AJR Am J Roentgenol 1991;157(2):249–53.

81. Kowal LE, Goodman LR, Zarro VJ, et al. CT diagnosis of broncholithiasis. J Comput Assist Tomogr 1983;7(2):321–3.

82. Shin MS, Ho KJ. Broncholithiasis: its detection by computed tomography in patients with recurrent hemoptysis of unknown etiology. J Comput Tomogr 1983;7(2):189–93.

Multidetector CT Evaluation of Tracheobronchomalacia

Edward Y. Lee, MD, MPH[a], Diana Litmanovich, MD[b],
Phillip M. Boiselle, MD[b],*

KEYWORDS

- Tracheomalacia
- Tracheobronchomalacia
- Bronchomalacia
- Multidetector computed tomography (MDCT)
- Clinical indications • Diagnostic criterion
- MDCT protocols • Image interpretation

Tracheobronchomalacia (TBM) is a disorder that results from a weakness of the tracheobronchial walls and/or supporting cartilage, resulting in excessive expiratory collapse (Fig. 1).[1–5] This condition may arise congenitally from disorders related to underlying impaired cartilage maturation or may be acquired from conditions related to prior intubation, infection, trauma, long-standing extrinsic central airway compression, or chronic inflammation.[1–5]

Although TBM has been increasingly recognized as an important cause of chronic respiratory symptoms, it is still considered a relatively under-diagnosed condition.[3] Because it escapes detection on routine end-inspiratory chest radiographs and CT scans, the diagnosis of TBM usually requires evaluating the airway during an active respiratory maneuver such as dynamic exhalation or coughing.[3,4,6] Recent advances in CT technology now allow the radiologist to accurately diagnose this condition noninvasively with similar accuracy to bronchoscopy, the historical reference standard.[6,7]

This article provides an up-to-date review of imaging for TBM, including clinical indications, physiologic principles, diagnostic criterion, multidetector CT (MDCT) protocols, multiplanar and 3-dimensional images, image interpretation, and pre- and postoperative assessment. An emphasis is placed on providing the reader with practical information that will enhance the ability to optimally perform and interpret CT studies for diagnosing TBM in daily clinical practice.

CLINICAL INDICATIONS

Although clinical indications have yet to be established for screening for TBM, the combination of chronic respiratory symptoms and one or more risk factors should raise the suspicion for this disorder. Risk factors for the acquired form of TBM are reviewed in Box 1.

It is important to be aware that extrinsic airway compression caused by paratracheal masses (such as mediastinal vascular anomalies and thyroid goiters) is frequently associated with tracheomalacia (TM) (Fig. 2).[3,8,9] For example, in children with paratracheal vascular anomalies such as innominate artery compression or vascular rings, surgical correction of the vascular anomalies alone may not adequately treat the respiratory symptoms if extrinsic compression is accompanied by intrinsic TM.[8,9] Thus, preoperative evaluation of

[a] Department of Radiology and Medicine, Children's Hospital Boston, Harvard Medical School, 300 Longwood Avenue, Boston, MA 02115, USA
[b] Department of Radiology, Center for Airway Imaging, Beth Israel Deaconess Medical Center, Harvard Medical School, Boston, MA 02115, USA
* Correspondence author.
E-mail address: pboisell@bidmc.harvard.edu (P.M. Boiselle).

Radiol Clin N Am 47 (2009) 261–269
doi:10.1016/j.rcl.2008.11.007
0033-8389/08/$ – see front matter © 2009 Elsevier Inc. All rights reserved.

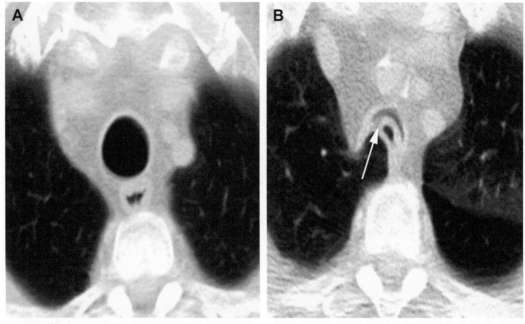

Fig. 1. CT diagnosis of TM in a 72-year-old man with shortness of breath. Paired inspiratory CT image (*A*) demonstrates a normal oval shape of the tracheal lumen. Dynamic expiratory CT image (*B*) shows excessive expiratory collapse of the trachea (*arrow*) consistent with TM.

such patients should routinely include a dedicated expiratory sequence to assess for TM.

Although pulmonary function studies (PFTs) are potentially useful in evaluating a patient with suspected TBM, they are not diagnostic of this entity.[3] On forced expiratory spirograms, patients with TBM frequently show a characteristic "break" or notch in the expiratory phase of the flow-volume loop;[3] however, this pattern may also be seen in patients with emphysema without coexisting TBM. Thus, MDCT is still necessary for confirming and characterizing TBM in such patients.

PHYSIOLOGIC PRINCIPLES

Functional CT imaging for TBM requires acquiring imaging data either during or after a provocative maneuver such as expiration and coughing. In order to understand why certain respiratory maneuvers are more effective than others at eliciting tracheal collapse, it is important to review the relationship of tracheal collapse to intrathoracic pressures. Changes in size of malacic trachea and bronchi depend on the difference between the intraluminal pressure inside the airways and the pleural (intrathoracic) pressure outside.[4,10] Pleural pressure depends mostly on respiratory muscles, and is high during expiratory efforts. In contrast, intraluminal pressures are highly variable, and depend on airflow. When airflow is zero, intraluminal pressure equals alveolar pressure and differs from pleural pressure only by the elastic recoil pressure of the lung, which depends on lung volume. At maximal lung volume with no flow (end-inspiration), the intraluminal pressure is 20 to 30 cm H_2O greater than pleural pressure, and the pressure difference expands the trachea.

Box 1
Risk factors for acquired tracheomalacia

Chronic obstructive pulmonary disease

Iatrogenic

  Prior intubation

  Prior tracheostomy

  Radiation therapy

  Lung transplantation

Chronic bronchitis

Relapsing polychondritis

Chest trauma

Chronic external compression of the trachea

  Paratracheal neoplasms (benign and malignant)

  Paratracheal masses (eg, goiter, congenital cyst)

  Aortic aneurysms and vascular rings

  Skeletal abnormalities (eg, pectus, scoliosis)

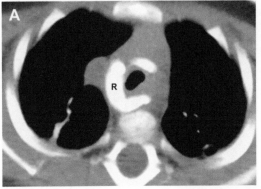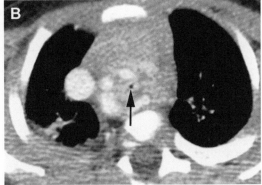

Fig. 2. TM in a young child associated with extrinsic compression from mediastinal vascular anomaly. Inspiratory contrast-enhanced CT image (*A*) demonstrates mild tracheal compression from a right-sided aortic arch (R) with aberrant left subclavian artery. Dynamic expiratory CT image (*B*) at similar level demonstrates near collapse of the trachea (*arrow*), consistent with severe TM. Prominent thymic tissue is noted in the mediastinum, consistent with the patient's young age.

At low lung volumes with no flow (end-expiration), the intraluminal pressure is nearly equal to pleural pressure, and the trachea is unstressed. The trachea is most compressed during cough and dynamic expiration at low lung volume, when pleural pressure is high ($\sim$100 cm H_2O), and expiratory flow limitation in the small airways prevents transmission of the high alveolar pressures to the central airways. Under these conditions, intraluminal pressure is nearly atmospheric, and the large transmural pressure causes tracheal collapse.[4,10]

Thus, based on physiologic principles, imaging during a forced exhalation or coughing maneuver is more sensitive for eliciting TBM than imaging at end-expiration.

DIAGNOSTIC CRITERION

Although greater than 50% expiratory reduction in cross-sectional area of the airway lumen is widely considered diagnostic of TM, it is important to be aware that asymptomatic, healthy individuals may demonstrate levels of expiratory collapse that exceed this diagnostic threshold (Fig. 3). For example, Stern and colleagues[11] obtained a degree of tracheal collapse greater than 50% at end-expiration in 4 of 10 healthy young adult male volunteers scanned with an electron-beam CT. Based on their findings, these authors recommended a more conservative threshold of 70% of collapse as indicative of TM. Similarly, Heussel and colleagues[12] reported that healthy volunteers can sometimes exceed the standard diagnostic criterion. Moreover, when using 64-MDCT "cine" imaging to assess the trachea during coughing, it has been suggested that a higher threshold value of 70% should be considered when using this

robust provocative maneuver to elicit tracheal collapse.[13]

Based on the results of these studies, there is a need to obtain normative data regarding the range of tracheal collapse using forced exhalation among patients of varying ages, ethnicities, and both genders, both with and without coexistent pulmonary disease. Until such data are published, one should keep in mind that there is substantial overlap with normal physiologic changes at the lower range of positive results. Thus, MDCT results should be carefully correlated with respiratory symptoms and functional impairment.

MULTIDETECTOR CT TECHNIQUES

Three main types of MDCT techniques are currently used for evaluating TBM: (1) paired end-inspiratory and end-expiratory MDCT; (2) paired end-inspiratory and dynamic expiratory MDCT; and (3) cine MDCT combined with a coughing maneuver.

Paired End-Inspiratory/End-Expiratory Multidetector CT

With this method, inspiratory and expiratory phases of volumetric CT data acquisition are obtained at the end of inspiration and expiration, respectively. Because imaging at the end of expiration is the least sensitive method for eliciting expiratory collapse, this technique should be limited to the assessment of infants and children younger than 5 years of age who are unable to cooperate with dynamic expiratory breathing instructions. For such patients, end-inspiratory and end-expiratory phases of the CT scanning are obtained following intubation by alternatively applying and withholding positive pressure

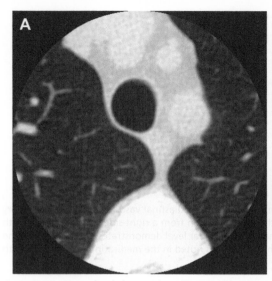
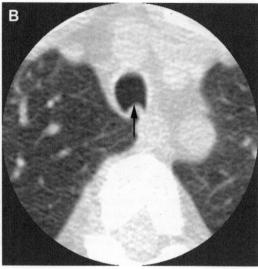

Fig. 3. Dynamic tracheal changes in a 45-year-old asymptomatic male volunteer with normal pulmonary function. Axial end-inspiratory CT image above level of aortic arch (*A*) demonstrates normal oval-shaped tracheal lumen. Axial dynamic-expiratory CT image at same level (*B*) demonstrates moderate anterior bowing of posterior membranous wall of trachea (*arrow*). Cross-sectional area of the tracheal lumen decreased by 51% during expiration, slightly exceeding the diagnostic criterion for TM.

ventilation during inspiration and expiration, respectively.[8,9] For detailed information about this method, the reader is referred to Lee and colleagues.[8,9]

Paired End-Inspiratory/Dynamic Expiratory Multidetector CT

This technique includes imaging during two different phases of respiration: end inspiration (imaging during suspended end inspiration) and continuous dynamic expiration (imaging *during* forceful exhalation). This protocol can be successfully performed with any type of MDCT scanner. However, the best results are produced with scanner configurations of eight or more detector rows.

At the authors' institutions, this technique is the method of choice for imaging adults and children older than 5 years for suspected malacia. In the following paragraphs, scanning parameters for imaging adults are reviewed. For detailed information about imaging children with this protocol, the reader is referred to Lee and colleagues.[8,9]

Before helical scanning, initial scout topographic images are obtained to determine the area of coverage, which extends from the proximal trachea through the main bronchi, corresponding to a length of approximately 10 to 12 cm in adults. If the patient has not had a recent CT scan, the end-inspiratory acquisition can be extended to

include the entire lungs to assess for potential complications of malacia such as bronchiectasis. Helical scanning is performed in the craniocaudal direction for both end-inspiratory and dynamic-expiratory scans.

The end-inspiratory scan is performed first (170 mAs, 120 kVp, 2.5 mm collimation, pitch equivalent of 1.5). Following the end-inspiratory scan, patients are subsequently coached with instructions for the dynamic expiratory component of the scan (40 mAs, 120 kVp, 2.5 mm collimation, high-speed mode, with pitch equivalent of 1.5). For this sequence, patients are instructed to take a deep breath in and to blow it out *during* the CT acquisition, which is coordinated to begin with the onset of the patient's forced expiratory effort. Detailed "scripts" of breathing instructions for this protocol can be found in an article by Bankier and colleagues.[14]

Cine CT During Coughing

This technique requires use of a 64-row or greater MDCT scanner. At the authors' institution this protocol is performed with detector collimation 0.5 mm × 64; mA = 80; kVp = 120; gantry rotation = 0.4 seconds.

An initial scout topographic image is obtained to determine the area of coverage, which extends 3.2 to 4.0 cm in craniocaudad length depending on the scan manufacturer. In order to "sample" the trachea and proximal main bronchi within a single acquisition, the inferior aspect of the acquisition is set at the level of the carina, and the superior aspect of the acquisition is set 3.2 cm above this level, which corresponds to approximately the level of the aortic arch in most adults. A 3- to 5-second acquisition is acquired in cine mode beginning at end-inspiration and followed by repeated coughing maneuvers. Images are reconstructed at 8-mm collimation in a standard algorithm, creating four contiguous cine datasets from a single acquisition.

The recently introduced dynamic-volume 320 MDCT scanner (Aquilion ONE, Toshiba Medical Systems) provides 16 cm of anatomic coverage in a single rotation.[15] This technique holds great promise for evaluating TBM because it provides coverage of the entire intrathoracic trachea in most older children and adults.

Radiation Exposure

Because paired inspiratory-expiratory CT requires imaging during two phases of respiration, it has the potential to result in a "double dose" compared with a traditional single-phase CT scan unless methods for dose reduction are used. Cine imaging also has the potential for high radiation exposure.

Because of the high inherent contrast between the air-filled trachea and soft tissue structures, it is possible to substantially reduce dose without negatively influencing image quality for assessing luminal dimensions of the airway.[4,6] For example, a clinical study by Zhang and colleagues[16] showed no difference between standard (240 to 260 mA) and low-dose (40 to 80 mA) images for assessing the tracheal lumen during dynamic expiration.

Thus, a low-dose (30 to 40 mAs) technique should be used when imaging during coughing or expiration. Although a standard mAs level is typically used for the end-inspiratory scan, dose modulation can be used to modify the mAs level during the acquisition to further reduce radiation exposure.

The estimated radiation dose (expressed as dose-length product) for a dual-phase study (standard-dose end-inspiratory sequence + low-dose dynamic expiratory sequence) for a 70-kg patient is approximately 500 mGy.cm, which is comparable to a routine chest CT (reference value 600 mGy.cm).[17] By comparison, the estimated dose for a low-dose cine CT is approximately 200 to 220 mGy.cm. However, unlike the dual-phase scan, which covers the entirety of the central airways, a single cine acquisition covers only 3.2 to 4.0 cm in the z-axis (depending on the scanner

configuration). If repeated at multiple levels to provide similar coverage to the dual phase CT, the total dose for serial cine acquisitions would be greater than the dual-phase technique. Estimated doses for cine imaging of the airways using the new 320 MDCT scanner are not currently available, but careful attention to dose reduction methods will be important with this scanner to avoid excessive radiation exposure.

Image Quality

In order to ensure a high-quality study, technologists should be trained to coach and monitor patients as they perform the respiratory techniques. Technologists should also be trained to recognize the characteristic appearance of inspiratory and expiratory CT scans to ensure that the imaging sequences have been successfully performed during the appropriate respiratory maneuvers (see Fig. 1). For sites using these protocols for the first time, the radiologist should observe and monitor cases until the technologists have become comfortable coaching patients with these maneuvers.

ROLE OF MULTIPLANAR AND 3-DIMENSIONAL RECONSTRUCTIONS

Volumetric MDCT imaging allows for the creation of high-quality, three-dimensional (3D) reconstructions and multiplanar reformations (MPR), which have the potential to aid diagnosis and preoperative planning.[4,18–21] Virtual bronchoscopic images, which provide an intraluminal perspective similar to conventional bronchoscopy, are particularly helpful for assessing dynamic changes in the lumen of the main bronchi, which course obliquely to the axial plane and are not optimally evaluated by traditional axial CT images. External 3D reconstructions are valuable for displaying complex 3D relationships in patients with extrinsic paratracheal masses such as aortic vascular anomalies.

Paired end-inspiratory and dynamic-expiratory sagittal reformation images along the axis of the trachea are helpful for displaying the craniocaudad extent of excessive tracheal collapse during expiration (Fig. 4).[4]

IMAGE INTERPRETATION

Interpretation of CT images requires careful review and comparison of both end-inspiratory and dynamic-expiratory images.

End-inspiratory images provide important anatomic information about tracheal size, shape, and wall thickness, as well as the presence or absence of extrinsic masses compressing the

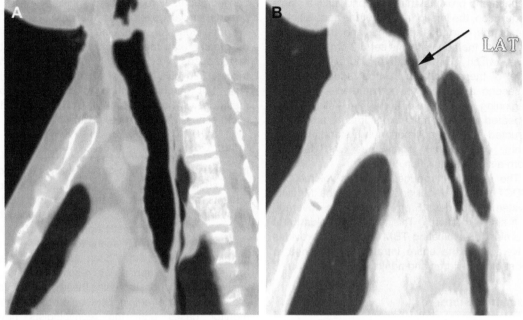

Fig. 4. Assessment of craniocaudad extent of TM in a 50-year-old woman with chronic cough. Paired end-inspiratory (A) and dynamic-expiratory (B) sagittal reformation images enhance display of craniocaudad length of TM. Note diffuse expiratory narrowing of trachea during expiration (B), consistent with diffuse TM.

trachea. In patients with TM, the tracheal lumen is almost always normal in appearance on end-inspiration CT.[2] There are four notable exceptions. First, patients with relapsing polychondritis (Fig. 5) frequently demonstrate characteristic wall thickening and calcification that spares the posterior membranous wall of the trachea. Second, patients with lunate (coronal > sagittal dimension) tracheal configurations (Fig. 6). Third, patients with tracheomegaly (coronal diameter > 25 mm). Fourth, patients with extrinsic tracheal compression from adjacent vascular anomalies or thyroid masses (see Fig. 2).

When there is near or complete collapse of the airway lumen during expiration, the diagnosis of malacia can be confidently made based on visual analysis of the images (see Fig. 1). However, the most accurate means for diagnosing malacia on CT in patients with subtotal expiratory collapse is to use an electronic tracing tool to calculate the cross-sectional area of the airway lumen on images at the same anatomic level obtained at inspiration and dynamic expiration (Fig. 7).[4] Such tools can be found on commercially available picture archiving and communication systems stations as well as with 3D workstations.

As described in the previous section, greater than 50% expiratory reduction in cross-sectional area is considered diagnostic. Care should be taken to

ensure that the same anatomic level is compared between the two sequences by comparing vascular structures and other anatomic landmarks.

Although quantitative methods are preferable to visual assessment, it is important to be aware that about half of patients with acquired TM will demonstrate an expiratory "frown-like" configuration, in which the posterior membranous wall is excessively bowed forward and parallels the convex contour of the anterior wall with less than 6-mm distance between the anterior and posterior walls (Fig. 8).[22] This appearance, which has been coined the "frown sign," has the potential to aid the detection of TM when patients inadvertently breathe during routine CT scans.[22]

With regard to interpreting cine coughing CT studies, these exams are ideally viewed in "cine" fashion at either a picture archiving and communication systems workstation or 3D workstation. Quantitative measurements are obtained on individual static images in a similar fashion to the technique described for paired-inspiratory–dynamic-expiratory CT. As described earlier, greater than 70% reduction in cross-sectional area during coughing is considered diagnostic. A commercial software program (Analyze 6.0, AnalyzeDirect, Inc., Lenexa KS) can also be used to provide automated measurement of changes in tracheal lumen cross-sectional area values during the cine sequence.[13]

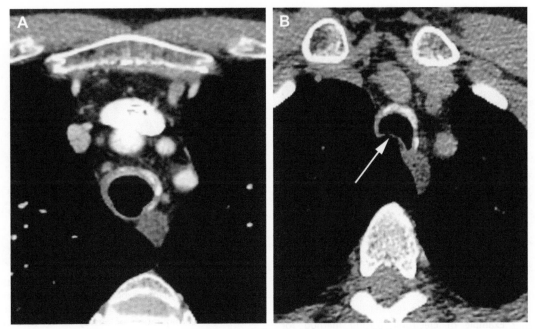

Fig. 5. TM in a 50-year-old woman with relapsing polychondritis presenting with intractable cough and dyspnea. End-inspiratory (*A*) and dynamic-expiratory (*B*) axial images of the upper trachea show calcified wall thickening with characteristic sparing of posterior membranous trachea. Excessive expiratory collapse of the trachea (*arrow*) is consistent with TM.

When interpreting functional CT scans of patients with TM, it is important to report the severity, distribution, and morphology. These factors have an important impact on treatment decisions, which are based on a combination of symptoms, severity and distribution of disease, and underlying cause of TM.[23]

Because there is not a single widely accepted scale for reporting the severity of TM, it is important to report the quantitative degree of

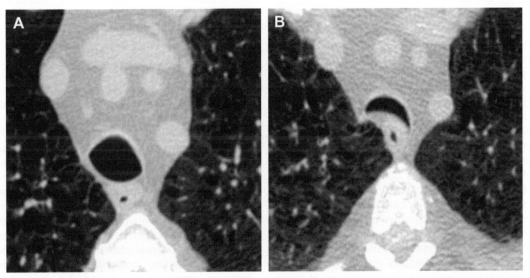

Fig. 6. Lunate configuration of the trachea in a 71-year-old woman with chronic cough and dyspnea. End-inspiratory CT image (*A*) demonstrates widening of coronal diameter of trachea with respect to the sagittal diameter, consistent with a lunate configuration. Dynamic-expiratory CT image (*B*) shows excessive expiratory collapse of airway lumen, consistent with TM.

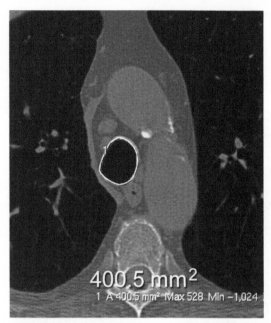

Fig. 7. Example of electronic tracing method for measuring cross-sectional area of tracheal lumen at the level of the aortic arch. The tracing line has been electronically thickened to enhance visibility for photographic reproduction. (*Reprinted from* Baroni RH, Feller-Kopman D, Nishino M, et al. Tracheobronchomalacia: comparison between end-expiratory and dynamic expiratory CT for evaluation of central airway collapse. Radiology 2005;235(2): 635–41; with permission.)

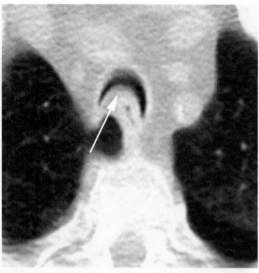

Fig. 8. "Frown sign" of TM in 64-year-old man with chronic cough. Dynamic expiratory CT image demonstrates excessive collapse of trachea with crescenteric, "frown-like" configuration of airway lumen (*arrow*), consistent with TM.

collapsibility rather than simply using a qualitative descriptor. A severity scale that has been used by some investigators includes three grades of severity based on the degree of airway collapse: (1) mild: 50% to 74%; (2) moderate: 74% to 99%; and (3) severe: 100% collapse.[7,23] In contrast, we consider more than 90% expiratory collapse as indicative of severe TM.

Murgu and Colt[23] recently proposed a functional class/extent/morphology/origin/severity (FEMOS) classification for TM. In this classification, a focal distribution of malacia is defined as involvement of one tracheal region (upper, middle, or lower) or involvement of one main or lobar bronchus. Multifocal distribution is defined as involvement of two contiguous or at least two noncontiguous regions, and diffuse involvement is defined as involvement of more than two contiguous regions. From a practical perspective, accurate determination of distribution has implications for treatment. For example, focal areas of malacia may benefit from stenting, whereas diffuse disease is more amenable to tracheoplasty surgery.

Regarding morphology, one should describe whether the collapse occurs circumferentially, or if it occurs primarily because of either excessive bulging of the posterior membranous wall or collapse of the anterolateral cartilaginous structures. For example, patients with collapse primarily because of bulging and flaccidity of the posterior membranous wall are potential candidates for tracheoplasty surgery, a novel surgical technique in which in the posterior wall of the trachea is reinforced by a Marlex graft.[24] Surgical reinforcement of the posterior membranous wall enhances the rigidity of this structure and makes it less susceptible to bowing during expiration.

PREOPERATIVE AND POSTOPERATIVE ASSESSMENT

CT plays several potentially important roles in evaluating severely symptomatic TM patients who are undergoing evaluation for curative tracheoplasty surgery.[24] Preoperative roles include (1) precise characterization of airway shape and determination of which parts of the airway wall contribute to excessive airway collapsibility; (2) evaluation for systemic diseases such as relapsing polychondritis that are not amenable to surgical therapy; (3) identification of extrinsic, paratracheal masses that may alter surgical planning; and (4) baseline measure of airway collapsibility by which to compare postoperative scans for evaluating response to surgery. In the postoperative setting, CT provides a noninvasive method for assessing for postoperative complications and noninvasively quantifying the degree of improvement in airway collapsibility.

Our surgeons and pulmonologists have found a combination of subjective symptomatic improvement and quantitative reduction in airway collapsibility at CT to be the most helpful measurements of determining response to surgery.[24] Our preliminary findings comparing preoperative and postoperative scans showed that tracheoplasty resulted in a decrease in the degree of airway collapse that was accompanied by a qualitative improvement of respiratory symptoms.[24]

SUMMARY

TBM refers to excessive expiratory collapse of the trachea and bronchi as a result of weakening of the airway walls and/or supporting cartilage. This disorder has recently been increasingly recognized as an important cause of chronic respiratory symptoms. MDCT technology allows for noninvasive imaging of TBM with similar accuracy to the historical reference standard of bronchoscopy. Paired end-inspiratory, dynamic expiratory MDCT is the examination of choice for assessing patients with suspected TBM. Radiologists should become familiar with imaging protocols and interpretation techniques to accurately diagnose this condition using MDCT.

REFERENCES

1. Paston F, Bye M. Tracheomalacia. Pediatr Rev 1996; 17:328.
2. Wright CD. Tracheomalacia. Chest Surg Clin N Am 2003;13:349–57.
3. Carden KA, Boiselle PM, Waltz DA, et al. Tracheomalacia and tracheobronchomalacia in children and adults: an in-depth review. Chest 2005;127:984–1005.
4. Boiselle PM. Tracheomalacia: functional imaging of the large airways with multidetector-row CT. In: Boiselle PM, White CS, editors. New techniques in cardiothoracic imaging. New York: Informa; 2007. p. 177–85.
5. Fraser RS, Colman N, Müller NL, et al. Upper airway obstruction. In: Fraser RS, Colman N, Müller NL, Pare PD, editors. Synopsis of diseases of the chest. 3rd edition. Philadelphia: BW Saunders; 2005. p. 631–4.
6. Lee KS, Sun ME, Ernst A, et al. Comparison of dynamic expiratory CT with bronchoscopy in diagnosing airway malacia. Chest 2007;131:758–64.
7. Gilkeson RC, Ciancibello LM, Hejal RB, et al. Tracheobronchomalacia: dynamic airway evaluation with multidetector CT. AJR Am J Roentgenol 2001;176:205–10.
8. Lee EY, Mason KP, Zurakowski D, et al. MDCT assessment of tracheomalacia in symptomatic infants with mediastinal aortic vascular anomalies: preliminary technical experience. Pediatr Radiol 2008;38:82–8.
9. Lee EY, Zurakowski D, Waltz DA, et al. MDCT evaluation of the prevalence of tracheomalacia in children with mediastinal aortic vascular anomalies. J Thorac Imaging 2008;23(4):258–65.
10. Baroni RH, Feller-Kopman D, Nishino M, et al. Tracheobronchomalacia: comparison between end-expiratory and dynamic expiratory CT for evaluation of central airway collapse. Radiology 2005;235(2):635–41.
11. Stern EJ, Graham CM, Webb WR, et al. Normal trachea during forced expiration: dynamic CT measurements. Radiology 1993;187(1):27–31.
12. Heussel CP, Hafner B, Lill J, et al. Paired inspiratory/expiratory spiral CT and continuous respiration cine CT in the diagnosis of tracheal instability. Eur Radiol 2001;11:982–9.
13. Boiselle PM, Lee KS, Lin S, et al. Cine CT during coughing for assessment of tracheomalacia: preliminary experience with 64-MDCT. Am J Roentgenol 2006;187(2):W175–7.
14. Bankier AA, O'Donnell C, Boiselle PM. Respiratory instructions for CT examinations of the lungs: a hands-on guideline. Radiographics 2008;28:919–31.
15. Johns Hopkins Installs First 320-slice CT scanner in North America. Johns Hopkins Medicine Web site. Available at: http://www.hopkinsmedicine.org/Press_releases/2007/11_26_07.html. November 26, 2007. Accessed July 28, 2008.
16. Zhang J, Hasegawa I, Feller-Kopman D, et al. Dynamic expiratory volumetric CT imaging of the central airways: comparison of standard-dose and low-dose techniques. Acad Radiol 2003;10:719–24.
17. Mayo JR, Aldrich J, Müller NL. Radiation exposure at chest CT: a statement of the Fleischner Society. Radiology 2005;228:15–21.
18. Boiselle PM, Reynolds KF, Ernst A. Multiplanar and three-dimensional imaging of the central airways with multidetector CT. Am J Roentgenol 2002;179:301–8.
19. Calhoun PS, Kuszyk B, Heath DG, et al. Three-dimensional volume rendering of spiral CT data: theory and method. RadioGraphics 1999;19:745–64.
20. Cody DD. Image processing in CT. RadioGraphics 2002;22:1255–68.
21. Lipson SA. Image reconstruction and review. In: Lipson SA, editor. MDCT and 3D workstations. 1st edition. New York: Springer Science + Business Media, Inc.; 2006. p. 30–40.
22. Boiselle PM, Ernst A. Tracheal morphology in patients with tracheomalacia: prevalence of inspiratory "lunate" and expiratory "frown" shapes. J Thorac Imaging 2006;21:190–6.
23. Murgu SD, Colt HG. Recognizing tracheobronchomalacia. J Respir Dis 2006;27:327–35.
24. Baroni RH, Ashiku S, Boiselle PM. Dynamic-CT evaluation of the central airways in patients undergoing tracheoplasty for tracheobronchomalacia. AJR 2005;184:1444–9.

Imaging–Bronchoscopic Correlations for Interventional Pulmonology

Tshering Amdo, MD[a], Myrna C.B. Godoy, MD[b],
David Ost, MD, MPH[c], David P. Naidich, MD, FACCP[b],*

KEYWORDS
- Interventional pulmonology • CT • Virtual bronchoscopy
- Endobronchial ultrasound (EBUS)
- Transbronchial needle aspiration (TBNA)

The development and rapid advancement of both bronchoscopic, CT and ultrasound imaging technology has had considerable impact on the management of a wide variety of pulmonary diseases. The synergy between these newer imaging modalities and advanced interventional endoscopic procedures has led to a revolution in diagnostic and therapeutic options in patients with both central and peripheral airway disease. Given the broad clinical implications of these technological advances, only the most important areas of interventional pulmonology in which imaging has had a major impact will be selectively reviewed to highlight fundamental principles.

Whereas interventional pulmonology is often conceptually organized around different technologies and instruments such as stents, lasers, and electrocautery, among others, it is important to emphasize applications of the same technology may vary widely in terms of their methods, risks, and benefits depending on the nature of the indication. For example, while the method in which a stent is placed may not alter, indications and complications are significantly different between patients with benign and malignant disease.[1] As a consequence, particular emphasis will be placed first on evaluation of CT-bronchoscopic correlations in the evaluation and treatment of central airway disease, followed by CT- bronchoscopic correlations in the evaluation of peripheral lung disease, in particular, pulmonary nodules. Following this, the rapidly evolving topic of interventional bronchoscopic approaches to the treatment of emphysema will be reviewed.

Although attention will be primarily be placed on CT bronchoscopic correlations (including CT-fluoroscopy and virtual bronchoscopy), emphasis will also be placed on newer imaging technologies including endobronchial ultrasound (EBUS), electromagnetic navigation and guidance, and Doppler ultrasound site selection for bronchoscopic treatment of emphysema.

BRONCHCOSCOPIC IMAGING CORRELATIONS IN THE EVALUATION OF CENTRAL AIRWAY DISEASE
CT Imaging Technique

Key to the recent ability of imaging to serve as a guide for interventional bronchoscopic procedures has been the introduction and now widespread availability of multidetector CT scanners capable of acquiring contiguous and/or overlapping high-resolution images throughout the entire thorax in a single breathhold. This has led to

[a] Division of Pulmonary and Critical Care Medicine, New York University–Langone Medical Center, Tisch Hospital, 560 First Avenue, New York, NY 10016, USA
[b] Department of Radiology, New York University–Langone Medical Center, Tisch Hospital 560 First Avenue, New York, NY 10016, USA
[c] Division of Pulmonary Medicine, MD Anderson Cancer Center, Houston, TX 77030, USA
* Corresponding author.
E-mail address: david.naidich@nyumc.org (D.P. Naidich).

Radiol Clin N Am 47 (2009) 271–287
doi:10.1016/j.rcl.2008.11.005

a near revolution in the variety of methods by which the airways and lung can be visualized and evaluated, including the use of quantitative CT techniques.[2,3] Although a truly detailed discussion of this topic is beyond the scope of the present review, the following general points regarding CT technique for evaluating the airways are emphasized.

Optimal evaluation of both the central and peripheral airways requires at a minimum contiguous high-resolution images throughout the entire chest (Fig. 1). While contiguous 1- to 1.5-mm sections are sufficient for evaluating both the central and peripheral airways, in our experience, optimal visualization of the peripheral airways is best obtained with use of submillimeter overlapping sections whenever possible (typically 0.75 mm every 0.5 mm) especially in those cases for which three-dimensional (3D) segmentation or virtual bronchoscopic evaluation of the peripheral (sixth to ninth order) airways is deemed clinically important.[4] Although the use of low-dose technique (50 to 80 mAs) is more than sufficient to evaluate the central airways and in most cases the peripheral airways as well, in those cases for which 3D and/or virtual endoscopic views are intended, best results necessitate the use of routine standard CT exposure factors. Additional considerations include acquisition of select expiratory high-resolution images in cases in which tracheal and bronchial dynamics are of concern, or to confirm the presence of obstructive small airway disease.

Axial CT images are sufficient for evaluating most airway abnormalities;[3,5] however, there are inherent limitations of these for assessing the central airways, including (1) limited ability to detect subtle airway stenosis; (2) underestimation of the craniocaudad extent of disease; (3) difficulty displaying the complex 3D relationships of the airway to adjacent mediastinal structures; (4) inadequate representation of airways oriented obliquely to the axial plane; and (5) difficulty assessing the interfaces and surfaces of airways that lie parallel to the axial plane. Another relative limitation of axial CT scanning is the generation of a large number of images for review, especially with multidetector scanners, which may generate data sets containing hundreds of images. As a consequence, use of retrospectively reconstructed 2D and 3D images should be considered routine for bronchoscopic correlation to overcome these limitations.

Virtual bronchoscopy (VB) in particular may facilitate central airway evaluation by allowing the user to "bypass" an obstructing lesion, accurately measure its length and cross-sectional area, and to look backward from distal to proximal, "retroflexing" the virtual bronchoscope, which is not possible with the conventional bronchoscope.[6] Virtual bronchoscopy is especially complementary to bronchoscopy in the assessment of patients with high-grade airway stenoses, particularly for assessing the patency of the airways beyond the site of a stenosis. In one study[7] comparing virtual and conventional bronchoscopy in 20 patients with malignant airway stenoses, while high-grade stenoses were viewed equally well with both techniques, virtual bronchoscopy offered the advantage of viewing the airway beyond the site of stenosis in 5 (25%) of 20 patients in whom the bronchoscope could not pass the lesion. However, lack of sensitivity for mucosal detail is an important limitation especially when attempting to assess the extent of airway wall involvement in patients in whom a distinction between intrinsic and extrinsic tumor is of clinical consequence.[6,8]

Finally, it is worth emphasizing that in those case in which there are central lesions accompanied by peripheral volume loss, administration of a bolus of intravenous contrast medium may prove indispensable by allowing precise delineation of the true extent of tumor versus atelectatic lung, findings often indispensable for selecting optimal therapeutic interventions.

Transbronchial Needle Aspiration and Biopsy

CT-bronchoscopic correlations

Transbronchial needle aspiration and biopsy (TBNA) is a minimally invasive procedure done via flexible fiber-optic bronchoscopy (FB) that allows sampling of tissue through the tracheal or bronchial wall not directly visualized bronchoscopically. TBNA was first introduced by Schieppati[9] in 1958 for use with the rigid bronchoscope and was later adapted for flexible bronchoscopy (FB) by Wang and colleagues in 1983.[10] This technique has been successfully used since then as a nonsurgical means most often to sample mediastinal nodes or less commonly hilar nodes, endobronchial lesions, and peripheral lesions for the diagnosis of both benign and neoplastic conditions.

The ability of TBNA to sample mediastinal and hilar nodes can reduce the need for invasive mediastinoscopy for assessing paratracheal lymph nodes and the need for open thoracotomy for posterior, subcarinal, and hilar lymph nodes, respectively.[11,12] Importantly, TBNA may provide the only bronchoscopic specimen diagnostic for lung cancer in up to 18% of patients in one reported series.[13] However, TBNA is often a "blind" procedure, especially when limited to sampling

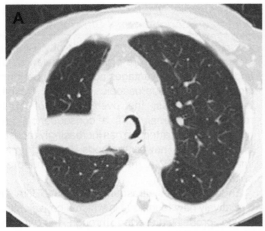 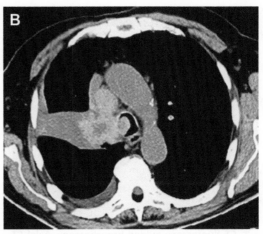

Fig. 1. Central airway lesions. (A) Section through the lower trachea imaged with lung windows shows a well-defined obstructing lesion. (B) Identical image as in A imaged with mediastinal window clearly demonstrates the true extent of tumor which appears denser then adjacent peripheral atelectasis. The ability to demonstrate the extent of tumor is critical to deciding the optimal method for interventional bronchoscopic therapy.

peribronchial lesions in the absence of endobronchial abnormalities. As a consequence, use of TBNA has been limited with an overall sensitivity for diagnosing malignant mediastinal adenopathy of 78% with values ranging from 14% to 100%.[14]

Although the sensitivity and specificity of TBNA largely depends on operator technique, the yield of TBNA has been shown to be markedly enhanced by using CT scans to plan optimal biopsy sites before bronchoscopy.[12,15] It should be emphasized, however, that merely identifying an enlarged node adjacent to a central airway on CT may not lead to successful TBNA, as not all endoscopic sites are equally amenable to transbronchial biopsy. As a consequence, optimal endoscopic anatomic landmarks for 14 hilar, intrapulmonary, and mediastinal lymph node stations have been proposed.[11] This classification provides for consistent, reproducible, lymph node mapping that is compatible with the international staging system for lung cancer[16] and is applicable for clinical and surgical-pathologic staging.

Whereas TBNA is most often performed to diagnose and stage NSCLC, it has also been used successfully to diagnose benign diseases as well, including, in particular, sarcoidosis[17] and more recently tuberculous lymphadenopathy in patients with HIV+/AIDS.[18] Especially in the setting of HIV+/AIDS, active tuberculous nodes may appear as rim-enhancing low-density lesions following intravenous contrast administration. In one series, using CT as a guide, mycobacterial infection was diagnosed by TBNA in 21 of 23 cases of documented mycobacterial infection, with TBNA providing the only diagnostic specimen in 13 (57%).[18]

CT fluoroscopic guidance

In 1998, Rong and Cui[19] demonstrated an increase in the yield by performing TBNA under CT guidance. Using conventional CT scanners to provide cross-sectional views of the relevant anatomy during the procedure, the tip of the needle was located and then adjusted until it was documented to be inside targeted mediastinal lymph nodes. Slow CT reconstruction times and significant radiation exposure, however, limit the practical value of this approach.

With the introduction of CT fluoroscopy, real-time imaging during the procedure became feasible enabling continuous image acquisition, permitting precise, real-time localization of the bronchoscopic tip and needle (Fig. 2). CT fluoroscopy is less cumbersome than conventional CT guidance, as it is controlled via a foot pedal with the imaging screen mounted next to the bronchoscopist obviating reliance on the technologist's workstation to check the position of the catheter tip. To date, several case series[20,21,22,23] have demonstrated the safety and ease of performing TBNA under CT fluoroscopic guidance with an increase in yield of diagnosis in patients previously undergoing nondiagnostic conventional TBNA.[20,21,23] White and colleagues[23] performed TBNA with CT fluoroscopic assistance on 27 patients, of whom 15 had mediastinal nodes and 12 had lung nodules or focal infiltrates. Mean lesion size was 1.7 cm in the mediastinum and 2.2 cm in the lung. A correct diagnosis was established in 10 of 12 mediastinal lesions (83%) for which follow-up was available (three patients were lost to follow-up) and in eight lung lesions (67%).[23] These investigators concluded that CT fluoroscopy

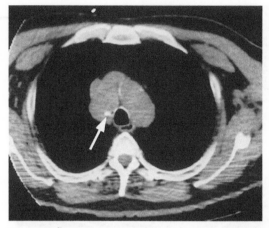

Fig. 2. CT fluoroscopy-guided bronchoscopy. Axial CT section through the distal trachea shows the tip of a TBNA needle in an enlarged right paratracheal lymph node (*arrow*), which on cytology proved to be due to metastatic non–small cell lung cancer. As demonstrated in this case, TBNA not only allows diagnosis, often the sole means for acquiring histologic diagnosis, but may also provide precise tumor staging—in this case Stage IIIA disease, obviating more invasive procedures including mediastinoscopy and/or surgery.

can provide effective, real-time guidance for TBNA and might be particularly valuable in patients with small or less accessible mediastinal nodes.[23]

Despite these results, a recent randomized trial failed to demonstrate a significant difference between CT fluoroscopic-guided bronchoscopy and conventional approaches, although this may reflect the small sample size of this study as there was a trend toward higher diagnostic yield with CT guidance on a per lymph node versus a per patient basis.[24] Finally, it should be noted that some have advocated the use of virtual bronchoscopic guidance as a means for enhancing the yield of TBNA (**Fig. 3**). Vining and colleagues[6] compared VB images with videotaped bronchoscopy results in 20 patients who had undergone both helical chest CT and FB during clinical evaluation of central airway abnormalities and observed that virtual bronchoscopy simulations accurately represented major endobronchial anatomic findings. As an extension of these findings, McAdams and colleagues[25] assessed the role of virtual bronchoscopy in guiding TBNA in 17 patients and found that it improved the diagnostic yield of this procedure, with an overall sensitivity of 88% on a per-node basis, and reduced both the amount of pre-procedure preparation and the actual procedural time. To date, while suggestive, an actual role for routine VB-guided TBNA remains to be established.

Transbronchial Needle Aspiration–Endobronchial Ultrasound

As discussed above, the yield of TBNA is clearly enhanced by pre-procedural review of CT findings: further advantages accrue from performing TBNA with fluoroscopic guidance. Despite these advantages, the overall yield of TBNA remains suboptimal.[14] As a consequence, and not surprisingly, attention has increasingly focused on developing newer methods for performing image-guided TBNA, most importantly endobronchial ultrasound.

Endobronchial ultrasound (EBUS)-TBNA is a relatively new technique in which a convex ultrasound probe is inserted through the working channel of the bronchoscope allowing real-time ultrasound-guided TBNA. After imaging the target lymph node, a specially designed TBNA needle is passed through the ultrasound catheter into the desired location under real-time ultrasound guidance (**Fig. 4**). EBUS-TBNA can be used to sample all except anterior, prevascular, and aorticopulmonary lymph nodes. This includes the highest mediastinal, upper and lower paratracheal, and subcarinal as well as hilar lymph nodes.[26,27,28] Compared with conventional TBNA, EBUS guidance significantly increases the yield of TBNA in all mediastinal lymph node locations except for subcarinal nodes.[29]

Of particular interest, EBUS has been shown to diagnose malignant mediastinal and hilar nodes in patients in whom both CT and positron emission tomography (PET) scans have proved negative.[30]

Similar findings have been reported by others. Yasufuku and colleagues,[31] for example, in a prospective comparison of EBUS-TBNA with PET and thoracic CT for detection of mediastinal and hilar lymph node metastasis in patients with lung cancer using surgical nodal sampling as a gold standard, showed that the sensitivities of CT, PET, and EBUS-TBNA for mediastinal and hilar lymph node staging were 76.9%, 80.0%, and 92.3%, respectively, with corresponding specificities of 55.3%, 70.1%, and 100%, and diagnostic accuracies of 60.8%, 72.5%, and 98.0%. Other investigators, however, have demonstrated that although EBUS may be useful in this situation, the frequency of occult mediastinal disease may be too low to make routine EBUS worthwhile. Cerfolio and colleagues[32] conducted a prospective trial on patients with NSCLC who were clinically staged N2 negative by both dedicated CT scanning and/or integrated PET/CT. All underwent mediastinoscopy and endoscopic ultrasonography (EUS) esophageal endoscopic ultrasound-guided fine-needle aspiration

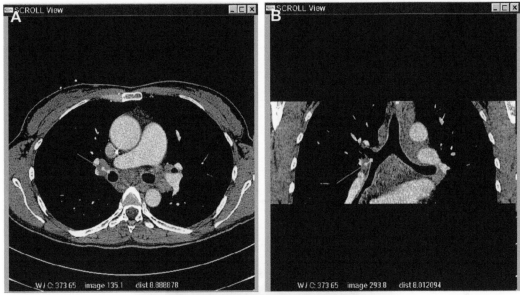

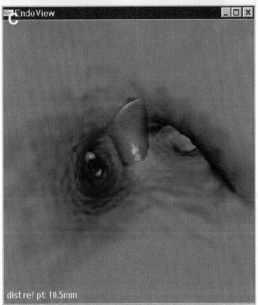

Fig. 3. TBNA: virtual bronchoscopic guidance. Axial (*A*) and coronal (*B*) CT sections imaged with narrow windows at the level of the bronchus intermedius show enlarged bilateral hilar and subcarinal nodes. In this case, right hilar nodes have been semiautomatically outlined and appear in color. Note that the optimal angle for accessing these nodes is also presented (*yellow lines*). (*C*) Virtual bronchoscopic image looking inferiorly from the distal bronchus intermedius showing the bifurcation of the right upper lobe bronchus and bronchus intermedius. The exact location of the right hilar nodes outlined in *A* and *B* are now superimposed on the virtual broncho-scopic image. In this case, virtual bronchoscopy serves as a road map assisting TBNA in accessing nodes in loca-tions less frequently biopsied. Cytologically proven metastatic non–small cell carcinoma. (*From* Naidich DP, Webb WR, Grenier PA, Harkin TJ, Gefter WB. Imaging the airways. Philadelphia: Lippincott Williams and Wilkins; 2005. p. 49; with permission.)

(FNA). Those with negative N2 nodes underwent thoracotomy with thoracic lymphadenectomy to confirm the findings. Only 2.9% of patients clini-cally staged as N0 after integrated PET/CT and/or CT had positive mediastinoscopy results and only 3.7% had positive EUS-guided FNA results. Based on these findings, these authors concluded that there was no indication for the use of routine EUS-guided FNA in patients with radiographic N0 disease. However, as patients with clinical

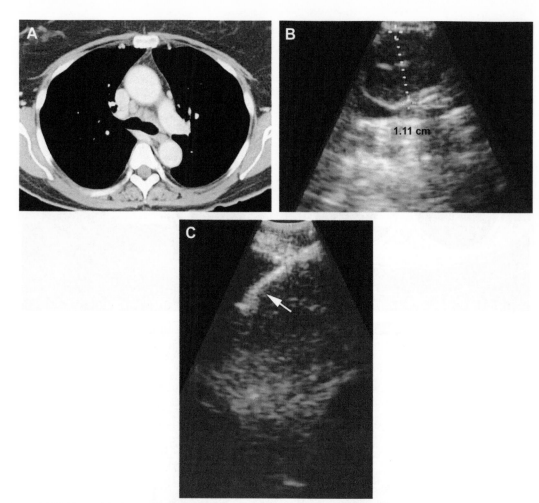

Fig. 4. EBUS-TBNA. (*A*) Contrast-enhanced axial CT image at the level of the carina shows slightly enlarged pre-carinal nodes. (*B*) Endobronchial ultrasound image shows these same nodes adjacent to the airway wall noted at the top of the image, measured at a depth of 1.1 cm. Nodes are especially easy to identify with EBUS separable from adjacent airways and vessels. (*C*) Endoscopic image confirming in real time that the TBNA needle tip is within the center of these nodes (*arrow*). Cytologically proven non–small cell lung cancer. (*Case courtesy of* Michael Zervos, MD, New York University–Langone Medical Center, New York NY.)

N1–hilar adenopathy by PET/CT had a relatively higher prevalence of unsuspected N2 disease (a total of 17.6% after mediastinoscopy and 23.5% after EUS-guided FNA) these investigators did conclude that patients with N1 disease be considered for routine EUS-FNA. Despite these findings, the need for preoperative EBUS-TBNA of otherwise normal-appearing mediastinal nodes remains to be determined.

Therapeutic Interventional Bronchoscopy: Imaging Correlations

The past decade has seen the development of a number of interventional bronchoscopic alternatives to routine therapeutic modalities for treating central airway disease. To date, these procedures are most often performed either as complementary to and/or alternatives to surgery, radiation, and/or chemotherapy in the palliative treatment of patients with malignant airway disease. Approximately 30% of lung cancer patients present with lesions obstructing either the trachea or main bronchi resulting in dyspnea, cough, hemoptysis, or symptoms secondary to obstructive pneumonia, especially when the degree of obstruction exceeds 50%.[33,34] Importantly, the ability to recanalize obstructed airways has proved of clinical benefit by alleviating symptoms and, in select cases, prolonging survival.

Currently available ablational procedures include Nd:YAG laser bronchoscopy, photodynamic therapy, argon plasma coagulation, endobronchial stents, brachytherapy, and cryosurgery.[35] Although a detailed description of these various procedures, including their mechanisms of action, is outside the intended scope of the present review, a few basic principles regarding their use warrant emphasis. Airway obstruction may result either from intrinsic tumor, extrinsic disease (typically from adjacent adenopathy, but also including other mediastinal malignancies) or a combination of these causes. In one study of 143 patients in whom stents were placed to alleviate obstruction, of 67% with malignant disease, 42% were because of extrinsic compression whereas 27% had intraluminal tumors.[36] Differentiation between these causes is of significance: stents and brachytherapy, for example, are best suited for extrinsic compression or in cases in which there is extensive submucosal disease (Fig. 5).[33] In distinction, in patients with intrinsic airway lesions, options preferentially include tumor debulking with the rigid bronchoscope, laser, cryotherapy, argon plasma coagulation, and photodynamic therapy (Fig. 6).[33] Among these latter, cryotherapy, photodynamic therapy, and brachytherapy are generally reserved for smaller endobronchial tumors where distal bronchial segments can be visualized[37] Although choice among these various approaches is individual depending on availability and technical expertise, in all cases CT may prove indispensable

by delineating the true extent of disease, both intrinsic and extrinsic, as well as allowing visualization of airways peripheral to points of obstruction otherwise invisible to the bronchoscopist.[3,38]

To date, CT has proved especially useful in the pre- and post-procedural assessment of airway stents. For airway stenting, routine 2D multiplanar reconstructions (MPRs) have proved of greatest utility clinically.[39] Easily obtained, MPRs can be displayed in routine coronal and sagittal planes, orthogonal to a point of reference, or in a curved fashion along the axis of the airway. The 2D reformatted images performed along the axis of the airway offer the advantage of quickly displaying the regional extent of a stenosis on a single image, although more difficult and time consuming to reconstruct.

As an aid, pre-procedural CT planning may prove invaluable by precisely delineating the anatomy, pathology, and severity of airway obstruction.[39] Information provided by CT can help to determine whether the airway obstruction is caused by extrinsic compression, intraluminal disease, or intrinsic airway disease, as occurs in patients with tracheobronchomalacia, for example.[40] CT also provides important complementary information regarding the relationship of the central airways to adjacent structures that are not visible at bronchoscopy.[39] By determining the cause, location, length, and extent of the airway obstruction, CT can help stratify patients

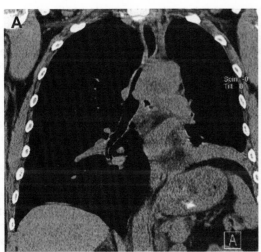 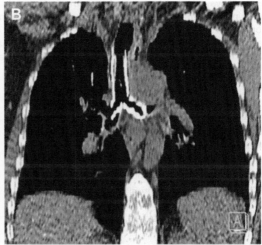

Fig. 5. Airway compression caused by extrinsic disease. (A) Non–contrast-enhanced multiplanar coronal reconstruction through the distal trachea and carina shows marked narrowing of these airways with apparent complete obstruction of the left mainstem bronchus resulting in marked volume loss in the left lung. (B) Coronal image at the same level as A showing the placement of a Y-shaped dynamic silicone stent in the distal trachea and proximal mainstem bronchi resulting in improved aeration of the left lung. Multiplanar reconstructions, in particular, facilitate identification of appropriate candidates for stenting as well as facilitating more precise measurement of airway diameter, lesion length, and airway visualization beyond the reach of the bronchoscope because of obstruction.

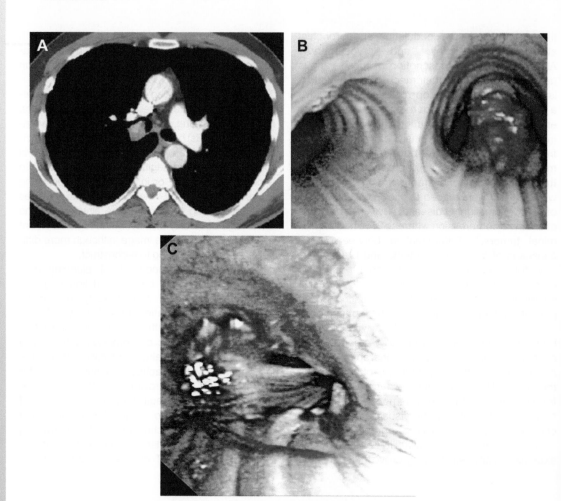

Fig. 6. Airway obstruction caused by intrinsic tumor. (*A*) Contrast-enhanced axial image just below the carina shows near complete obstruction of the right mainstem bronchus by a well-defined soft tissue mass. (*B*) Endoscopic view showing bulky tumor mass appearing to completely occlude the airway lumen. (*C*) Endoscopic view following photodynamic therapy documenting marked decrease in the size of this lesion, which proved to be a mucoepidermoid carcinoma. CT may play an invaluable role by demonstrating the true extent of disease allowing optimal choice of interventional technique.

into those who are amenable to surgical resection and those who are candidates for palliative treatment (see Fig. 5). In patients deemed appropriate for airway stenting, CT findings can help to determine the type, size, and length of stent needed. For cases in which the initial bronchoscopic evaluation fails to visualize the airways beyond the site of obstruction, CT serves as an important adjunct study by providing detailed anatomic information of the distal airways.[39]

Less common, although as important, indications for interventional bronchoscopic procedures include the treatment of benign tumors or a number of benign conditions, most often postintubation tracheal strictures. Gluecker and colleagues,[41] for example, compared 2D and 3D CT imaging in the pre- and postoperative evaluation of complex benign laryngeo-tracheal airway stenoses with rigid bronchoscopy, considered as the gold standard. Two-dimensional images and 3D VB of tracheal stenoses proved to be efficient and complementary to rigid bronchoscopy, permitting a reliable endoluminal 3D view and evaluation of the surrounding anatomic structures.

In addition to assisting in pre-procedural planning, CT is also being increasingly used as a first-line study for stent surveillance.[39,42] Because nearly all stents, including metallic stents, cause minimal artifact on multislice CT, the location, shape, and patency of the stents and adjacent airways can be clearly visualized on CT. CT is highly accurate at detecting stent complications, including malpositioning, migration, fracture, incongruence between the stent and airway diameters, external compression with continued stenosis, and local recurrence of malignancy

(Fig. 7). When compared with fiber-optic bronchoscopy, both MPRs and 3D renderings have been shown to be 88% to 100% sensitive and 100% specific in detecting stent complications.[42,43] In a recent study by Dialani and colleagues,[42] for example, CT accurately detected 15 (100%) of 15 stent complications in a group of patients undergoing surveillance with both CT and bronchoscopy leading these investigators to suggest that CT may be able to replace bronchoscopy for routine surveillance of stents.

Bronchoscopic Imaging Correlations for Peripheral Lesions

It has long been noted that the likely yield of transbronchial needle aspiration or biopsy (TBBx) of peripheral lung nodules or masses is affected by the size and location of lesions. Peripheral lesions (defined as those not visible bronchoscopically beyond the segmental bronchial level) in particular are problematic with sensitivities of 34% for peripheral lesions smaller than 2 cm in diameter versus 63% for lesions with a diameter larger than 2 reported in one recent study including 30 patients with peripheral lung lesions.[44] Additional factors include the type of lesion (solid versus groundglass), the type of procedure performed (bronchoalveolar lavage versus bronchial brushing versus TBBx), or whether the procedure is performed under fluoroscopic control.

The CT Bronchus Sign/CT Fluoroscopy

It has been shown that the likely yield of TBNA for peripheral lesions is significantly improved in those cases in which a bronchus can be identified leading to or traversing a nodule, a so-called "positive bronchus sign."[45,46] It has also been suggested that improved results from attempted transbronchial biopsy may result when CT fluoroscopy has been used to aid in the diagnosis of peripheral lesions (Fig. 8). To date, while there have been several small promising case series reported,[19,20,22,23,47] there has been only one small randomized controlled trial[24] comparing CT fluoroscopy–guided bronchoscopy with conventional bronchoscopy for the diagnosis of peripheral lesions. In this study, there was no significant difference between CT fluoroscopy–guided bronchoscopy and conventional bronchoscopy;[24] however, when CT confirmed entry of the biopsy forceps or needle into peripheral lesions, the diagnostic yield did prove considerably higher. This result suggests that the overall yield of CT-guided bronchoscopy could be considerably enhanced if combined with improved methods of steering, not only using conventional but ultrathin bronchoscopes as well.

In this regard, VB has recently been applied to aid in the diagnosis of peripheral lesions. Asano and colleagues[48] used VB and ultrathin bronchoscopy for peripheral pulmonary lesions. The diagnosis

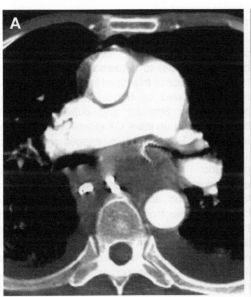 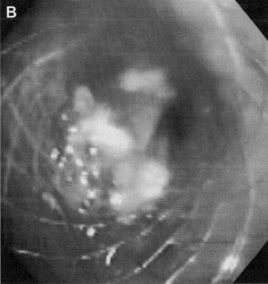

Fig. 7. Stent surveillance. (A) Enlargement of a contrast-enhanced axial CT image below the carina shows extensive mediastinal tumor associated with bilateral pleural effusions. Note that there is a stent seen in the left main stem bronchus within which soft tissue density is clearly identifiable, in this case because of tumor invasion of the stent. CT is an effective means for monitoring stents following placement. (B) Endoscopic view confirming tumor infiltrating the lumen through the stent.

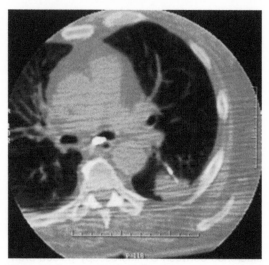

Fig. 8. CT fluoroscopy: peripheral lung disease. Axial non–contrast-enhanced image obtained during fluoroscopic-guided transbronchial biopsy. Note that images obtained during CT fluoroscopy suffer from some degree of motion artifact and increased image noise. In this case it is possible to identify the tip of the biopsy needle within the center of a lesion in the superior segment of the left lower lobe. Cytologically proven non–small cell lung cancer.

rate of this procedure was 81.6% for the 38 lesions examined by ultrathin bronchoscopy: 80.8% for 26 lesions 2 cm in size, and 83.3% for 12 lesions larger than 2 cm. Merritt and colleagues[49] and Shinagawa and colleagues[50] have also demonstrated that combining VB and ultrathin bronchoscopy was superior to conventional bronchoscopy for diagnosing peripheral lung lesions. Asahina and colleagues[51] successfully performed transbronchial biopsy (TBB) using EBUS and VB navigation for small peripheral pulmonary lesions smaller than 3 cm in diameter.

Despite these findings, it should be noted that currently available biopsy forceps for use in ultrathin bronchoscopes present an important barrier to the use of this approach, as only minimal tissue can generally be obtained, severely limiting diagnostic efficacy. More promising is the potential use of VB-guided bronchoscopy to precisely direct a pediatric bronchoscope into the lung periphery to sample specific regions in patients with otherwise "diffuse" lung diseases identified on high-resolution CT (HRCT).[4]

Endobronchial ultrasound with radial probe
EBUS using a radial ultrasonic probe has also been used to locate peripheral parenchymal lesions.[52] For this purpose a thin ultrasonic probe is inserted through a guide sheath that is passed

through the working channel of a flexible bronchoscope (FB). Under fluoroscopic guidance, the whole unit is maneuvered to the region of interest. Although the radial probe provides cross-sectional images of the tracheobronchial wall and adjacent mediastinal structures and produces a 360-degree image relative to the long axis of the FB, a major limitation has been the necessity to withdraw the US probe before inserting a biopsy instrument, eliminating the possibility of real-time positioning.

Paone and colleagues[53] conducted a study to compare the diagnostic yield of two bronchoscopic procedures: EBUS transbronchial biopsy (EBUS-TBB) and conventional transbronchial biopsy (TBB) for diagnosing peripheral pulmonary lesions and reported a sensitivity of 79% in the EBUS group versus 55% in the TBB group for establishing malignant diagnoses. In patients with lesions smaller than 3 cm, they found a considerable decline in TBB sensitivity and accuracy (31% and 50%), whereas EBUS-TBB maintained its diagnostic yield (75% and 83%). A similar difference in sensitivity was observed when lesions smaller than 2 cm (23% versus 71%) were compared. Based on these data it may be concluded that in select cases EBUS using a radial probe represents an important option in the diagnosis of peripheral lung cancer, especially in small lesions and/or patients considered ineligible for surgery.

Electromagnetic navigation
The electromagnetic navigation system is an image-guided localization device that assists in placing endobronchial accessories (forceps, brush, or needle) to desired regions of the lung (Fig. 9). The use of this novel technology in animal models followed by human subjects was first published by Schwarz and colleagues.[54,55] In brief, following an initial CT examination requiring contiguous 1-mm sections, images are then uploaded into a navigating computer. The electromagnetic navigation system creates an electromagnetic field around the chest by placing the subject on an electromagnetic localization board. An electromagnetic position sensor is then attached to the same navigating computer already loaded with the initial CT scan data, now displayed in virtual bronchoscopic format. As the sensor is positioned within the electromagnetic field, precise spatial coordinates are fed to the computer in real time and correlated with the virtual bronchoscopic CT data by a process of registration. This involves selecting predetermined targets on the virtual bronchoscopic image and then touching the corresponding identical

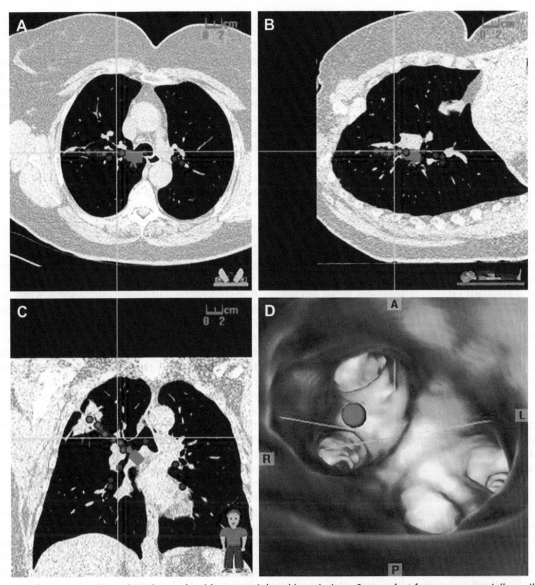

Fig. 9. Electromagnetic registration and guidance: peripheral lung lesions. Screen shot from a commercially available electromagnetic navigation system (SuperDimension, Inc) shows typical interface with axial, sagittal, and coronal CT images, respectively, coupled with virtual bronchoscopic images. Following an initial CT study, data are loaded into the navigating computer. Using virtual bronchoscopy (*lower right image*), anatomic landmarks are chosen as registration points. Typically these are the main carina, right upper lobe carina, middle lobe carina, right lower lobe carina, left upper lobe carina, and left lower lobe carina displayed in this image as purple dots. During actual bronchoscopy, the electromagnetic sensor is touched to each of these points enabling electronic registration of these locations by the computer. A separate path to the target lesion of interest (*green dots*) is also reconstructed. Once the registration process is complete, the bronchoscopist pilots from green dot to green dot until the target lesion is reached.

endoscopic targets in real time using the bronchoscopic probe. Targets chosen are points of airway bifurcation and include the main carina and most proximal lobar bifurcations. Once five to six of these anatomic locations have been so co-registered with the corresponding VB images, the computer can then map the rest of the CT data to real-life coordinates (see **Fig. 9**). Divergence, a measure of the error between the projected coordinates using these registration points and the actual points, is usually in the range of 3 to 7 mm.

Importantly, the electromagnetic navigation system includes two critical features. The electromagnetic position sensor, which is the size of a bronchoscopy forceps, first is steerable and second may be passed through an extended working channel, which is simply a hollow catheter. Consequently, once the probe reaches its intended target, it can be removed while keeping the extended working channel in place. Biopsy instruments such as forceps and brushes can then be passed back down the extended working channel to the same location.

Schwarz and colleagues[54,55] successfully demonstrated, initially in animal models and subsequently in a human study, safe use of electromagnetic navigation technology coupled with preoperative CT scanning in precisely localizing peripheral lung lesions with a variety of endobronchial accessories. They also demonstrated safety and efficacy in navigating to peripheral lung lesions located beyond the range of a standard FB.[54,55] Subsequent larger studies in human subjects[56,57,58,59] have been conducted with reproducible results, proving that electromagnetic navigation bronchoscopy is a safe method for sampling peripheral and mediastinal lesions with high diagnostic yield independent of lesion size and location. Nonetheless, despite the potential of widespread clinical applicability, it should be emphasized that, to date, no randomized trials demonstrating its superiority to conventional methods for diagnosing peripheral lung lesions has been reported.

Electromagnetic navigation plus endobronchial ultrasound

Although both EBUS using radial probes and electromagnetic navigation bronchoscopy have been used individually to try to improve bronchoscopic diagnosis of peripheral lung lesions, a recent study by Eberhardt and colleagues[60] evaluated whether or not the combination of radial EBUS plus electromagnetic navigation might be superior to either system alone. Focusing on the diagnosis of peripheral lung lesions, this study included three arms: EBUS only, an electromagnetic navigation system only, and a combined procedure using both technologies together. In the combined group, following initial electromagnetic navigation, an ultrasound probe was passed through the extended working channel to enable direct visualization of lesions. Biopsies were taken if ultrasound visualization confirmed that the extended working channel was within the target with retargeting of lesions performed as necessary. For the purpose of this study, primary outcome was defined as diagnostic yield with the reference standard surgical biopsy if bronchoscopic biopsy proved nondiagnostic. The diagnostic yield of the combined procedure (88%) was greater than EBUS (69%) or electromagnetic navigation (59%) alone, and proved independent of lesion size or lobar distribution. Based on this initial study, it was concluded that combining EBUS and electromagnetic navigation can improve the sensitivity of flexible bronchoscopy when compared with either EBUS or electromagnetic navigation individually for diagnosing peripheral lung lesions without compromising safety.[60] Similarly improved results using a combined approach have also been reported.[61]

Emphysema: CT-Interventional Bronchoscopic Correlations

Bronchoscopic lung volume reduction in severe emphysema

Current treatment of severe emphysema is limited to palliative measures that include supplemental oxygen, bronchodilators, anti-inflammatory drugs, and pulmonary rehabilitation or lung transplantation. Various surgical procedures have been used to treat severe emphysema, including thoracoplasty, excision of bullae, costochondrectomy, phrenic nerve division, autonomic denervation, and lung transplantation. Until the completion of the National Emphysema Treatment Trial (NETT),[62] none of these techniques were accepted as beneficial except for resection of giant bullae and lung transplantation, each indicated in only a small percentage of emphysema patients. The NETT trial established that Lung Volume Reduction Surgery (LVRS) is associated with improvement in health status, dyspnea, and exercise capacity and lung function, when compared with medical treatment in select populations.[62,63] In this regard, the extent and severity of disease as identified by CT has proved one of the most important predictors of a successful outcome, with patients with predominant upper lobe centrilobular disease most likely to respond successfully (Fig. 10), while those with more diffuse disease are noncandidates. However, because LVRS is associated with significant morbidity, mortality, and cost, nonsurgical alternatives for achieving volume reduction are being developed.

To date, three bronchoscopic lung volume reduction strategies have shown promise and are currently entering into clinical trials. All are designed to reduce hyperinflation within emphysematous portions of the lung and thus achieve lung volume reduction without the significant mortality and morbidity associated with surgical LVRS.[64,65,66,67] These include (1) placement of endobronchial one-way valves designed to promote

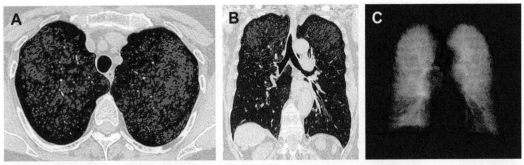

Cluster	Left				Right			
	Total	Upper	Middle	Lower	Total	Upper	Middle	Lower
Class 1 [%]	0.6	0.7	1.1	0.1	0.6	0.7	0.9	0.2
Class 2 [%]	0.6	0.7	1.1	0.0	0.7	1.0	0.9	0.1
Class 3 [%]	0.1	0.2	0.2	0.0	0.1	0.1	0.2	0.0
Class 4 [%]	9.1	23.8	3.3	0.0	6.6	6.6	1.8	0.1
3D BI []	4.6	4.7	4.3	0.0	4.6	4.6	2.6	0.2

Fig. 10. Emphysema: quantitative CT evaluation. Axial (A, upper left image), coronal (B, middle image), and volumetric rendered coronal sections (C, upper right image) show typical appearance of severe centrilobular emphysema almost exclusively restricted to the upper lobes. In this case, contiguous 1-mm images were acquired with quantitative analysis using −950 HU as a cut-off to demonstrate emphysematous foci, visually color-coded. The table below the images shows quantitative assessment of the extent of emphysema as measured by the so-called "cluster" analysis. This allows evaluation of the relative size of low-density foci providing a "bulla index" (3d BI) in which voxels are subdivided as in this example into four arbitrary classes, each separately color coded, with class 1 (blue) = all low-density foci ≤ 2 mm; class 2 (green) = 2 to 8 mm; class 3 (yellow) = 8 to 12 mm; and class 4 (pink) = 12 mm, respectively. Note that in this case the majority of low-density foci fall into the class 4 category and are clearly upper lobe in distribution without evidence of discrete subpleural bullae noted—findings ideal for both LVRS and/or bronchoscopic lung volume reduction.

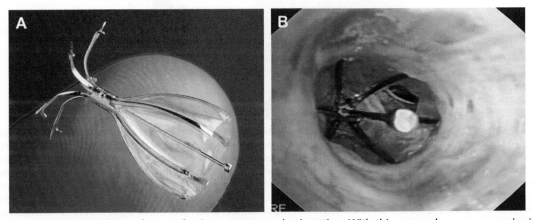

Fig. 11. Bronchoscopic lung volume reduction—one-way valve insertion. With this approach, a one-way valve is inserted under endoscopic guidance in an upper lobe bronchus to block air from entering the emphysematous portion of on inspiration while allowing gas to exit during expiration. (A) The appearance of the valve before insertion against the background of a person's finger. (B) The appearance of the valve 1 month following deployment within the right upper lobe bronchus, follow-up 9 months later showed marked narrowing of the right upper lobe bronchus consistent with marked volume loss in the right upper lobe.

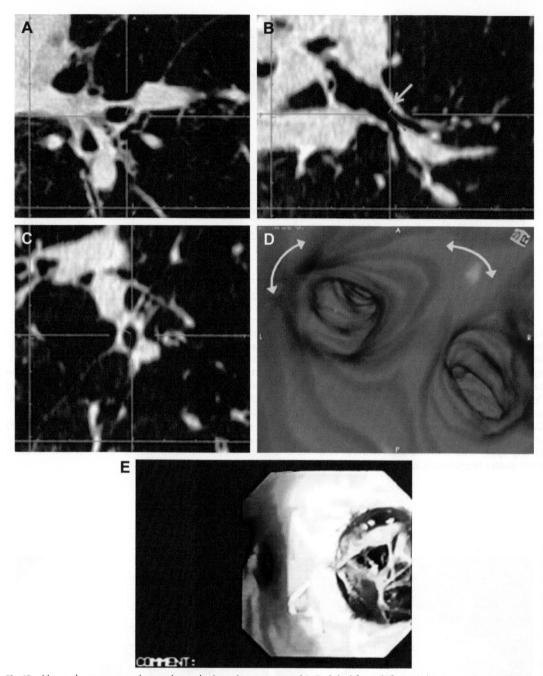

Fig. 12. Airway bypass procedure—drug-eluting airway stents. (*A–D, label from left to right, top to bottom*) Select coned down views of the proximal left lower lobe basilar bronchi in a patient with diffuse emphysema. CT scans are used not only to assess the severity and distribution of emphysema but also to identify blood vessels that need to be avoided during stent placement. With this approach, all lobes except the middle lobe are potential targets for intervention. Drug-eluting airway stents are placed in segmental airways leading to regions with the highest residual volume with the expectation that these will facilitate the escape of trapped air. Virtual bronchoscopic images are also used to further assist in determining optimal stent placement (*lower right image*). (*E*) Endoscopic view showing the appearance of the airway following stent placement. Note that the stent leads directly from a segmental airway to more distal respiratory bronchioles and alveoli.

atelectasis by blocking inspiratory flow; (2) formation of airway bypass tracts using drug eluting stents designed to facilitate emptying of "damaged" regions of the lung defined by long expiratory times; and (3) instillation of biological adhesives designed to collapse and remodel hyperinflated lung.[64,65,66,67]

For any of these techniques to work, careful delineation of the extent and type and severity of emphysema is essential.[68] Imaging therefore plays a pivotal role in bronchoscopic treatment of emphysema, because it facilitates measurement of the extent and distribution of emphysema as well as identifying concomitant conditions that either require additional evaluation (such as presence of associated severe bronchial disease, concomitant interstitial fibrosis, or potentially malignant lung nodules) that may represent contraindications to routine LVRS. Finally, delineation of airway anatomy relative to adjacent foci of emphysema may aid in the bronchoscopic procedure itself.

Currently, two endobronchial one-way valve systems are currently under evaluation.[64,65,66,67] Both are intended primarily for treatment of heterogeneous upper lobe emphysema again initially identified preferentially using quantitative CT scan data (Fig. 11). They are designed to block air from entering the target area during inspiration while allowing gas to exit during expiration with the intention of causing partial or preferably complete lobar collapse resulting in deflation of previously hyperinflated areas of the damaged lung. This allows improved ventilation because of expansion of the less extensively or uninvolved middle and especially lower lobes.

In airway bypass systems,[64,65,66,67] CT images are scored pre-procedure with the extent and severity of emphysema quantified using a variety of software programs currently available in a manner consistent with definitions established in the NETT trial.[62,68] Each lobe of the lung, except the middle lobe, is assessed independently and assigned a grade of 0, 1, 2, 3, or 4 based on the percentage of lung destruction within the lobe. After careful assessment of the pre-procedure CT data and airway anatomy by FB (Fig. 12), drug-eluting airway bypass stents are then placed in segmental airways leading to regions with the highest residual volume. This allows escape of excessive trapped gas by the creation of extra-anatomic passages.

SUMMARY

The improvements to patient care that can be achieved by combining advanced imaging techniques and bronchoscopy are considerable. In this regard, CT imaging often plays an indispensable role in both the selection of appropriate candidates for therapy as well as the choice of optimal interventional techniques. However, it is apparent that alternate methods for evaluating the airways and lung including ultrasound and electromagnetic navigation will likely play an increasingly important diagnostic role, necessitating a thorough understanding of their advantages and limitations. Disease-specific applications for which imaging technologies, including CT and VB, are either currently routinely used or show the greatest promise are for suspected or diagnosed lung cancers, central and peripheral, and emphysema. It may be anticipated that with growing experience, the potential for additional indications of these remarkable technologies are likely to increase in the near future.

REFERENCES

1. Chin CS, Litle VR, Yun J, et al. Airway stents. Review. Ann Thorac Surg 2008;85:S792–6.
2. Naidich DP, Gruden JF, McGuinness G, et al. Volumetric (helical/spiral) CT (VCT) of the airways. J Thorac Imaging 1997;12:11–28.
3. Grenier PA, BeigelmanAubry C, Fetita C, et al. Multidetector-row CT of the airways. Semin Roentgenol 2003;38:146–57.
4. Godoy MC, Ost D, Geiger B, et al. Utility of virtual bronchoscopy-guided transbronchial biopsy for the diagnosis of pulmonary sarcoidosis: report of two cases. Chest 2008;134:630–6.
5. Naidich DP, Lee JJ, Garay SM, et al. Comparison of CT and fiberoptic bronchoscopy in the evaluation of bronchial disease. AJR Am J Roentgenol 1987;148: 1–7.
6. Vining DJ, Liu K, Choplin RH, et al. Virtual bronchoscopy: relationships of virtual reality endobronchial simulations to actual bronchoscopic findings. Chest 1996;109:549–53.
7. Fleiter T, Merkle EM, Aschoff AJ, et al. Comparison of real-time virtual and fiberoptic bronchoscopy in patients with bronchial carcinoma: opportunities and limitations. Am J Roentgenol 1997;169:1591–5.
8. Finkelstein SE, Schrump DS, Nguyen DM, et al. Comparative evaluation of super high-resolution CT scan and virtual bronchoscopy for the detection of tracheobronchial malignancies. Chest 2003;124: 1834–40.
9. Schieppati E. Mediastinal lymph node puncture through tracheal carina. Surg Gynecol Obstet 1958;107:243–6.
10. Wang KP, Brower R, Haponik EF, et al. Flexible transbronchial needle aspiration for staging of bronchogenic carcinoma. Chest 1983;84:571–6.

11. Harkin TJ, Wang K-P. Bronchoscopic needle aspiration of mediastinal and hilar lymph nodes. J Bronchology 1997;4:238–49.

12. Wang K-P. Staging of bronchogenic carcinoma by bronchoscopy. Chest 1994;106:588–93.

13. Harrow EM, Abi-Saleh W, Blum J, et al. The utility of transbronchial needle aspiration in the staging of bronchogenic carcinoma. Am J Respir Crit Care Med 2000;161:601–7.

14. Detterbeck F, Janakiev D, Wallace M, et al. Invasive mediastinal staging of lung cancer: ACCP evidence-based clinical practice guidelines. (2nd Edition). Chest 2007;132:202S–20S.

15. Silvestri GA, Gould MK, Margolis M, et al. Noninvasive staging of non-small cell lung cancer: ACCP evidence-based clinical practice guidelines. (2nd Edition). Chest 2007;132:S178–201.

16. Mountain CF, Dresler CM. Regional lymph node classification for lung cancer staging. Chest 1997;111:1718–23.

17. Morales CF, Patefield AJ, Strollo PJ, et al. Flexible transbronchial needle aspiration in the diagnosis of sarcoidosis. Chest 1994;106:709–11.

18. Harkin TJ, Ciotoli C, Addrizzo-Harris DJ, et al. Transbronchial needle aspiration (TBNA) in patients infected with HIV. Am J Respir Crit Care Med 1998;157:1913–8.

19. Rong F, Cui B. CT scan directed transbronchial needle aspiration biopsy for mediastinal nodes. Chest 1998;114:36–9.

20. Garpestad E, Goldberg SN, Herth F, et al. CT fluoroscopy guidance for transbronchial needle aspiration an experience in 35 patients. Chest 2001;119:329–32.

21. Goldberg SN, Raptopoulos V, Boiselle PM, et al. Mediastinal lymphadenopathy: diagnostic yield of transbronchial meidastinal lymph node biopsy with CT fluoroscopic guidance. Initial experience. Chest 2000;216:764–7.

22. White CS, Templeton PA, Hasday JD, et al. CT-assisted transbronchial needle aspiration: usefulness of CT fluoroscopy. AJR Am J Roentgenol 1997;169:393–4.

23. White CS, Weiner EA, Patel P, et al. Transbronchial needle aspiration—guidance with CT fluoroscopy. Chest 2000;118:1630–8.

24. Ost D, Shah R, Anasco E, et al. A randomized trial of CT fluoroscopic-guided bronchoscopy vs. conventional bronchoscopy in patients with suspected lung cancer. Chest 2008;135:507–13.

25. McAdams HP, Goodman PC, Kussin P, et al. Virtual bronchoscopy for directing transbronchial needle aspiration of hilar and mediastinal lymph nodes: a pilot study. AJR Am J Roentgenol 1998;170:1361–4.

26. Yasufuku K, Chiyo M, Koh E, et al. Endobronchial ultrasound guided transbronchial needle aspiration for staging of lung cancer. Lung Cancer 2005;50:347–54.

27. Eloubeidi MA. Endoscopic ultrasound-guided fine-needle aspiration in the staging and diagnosis of patients with lung cancer. Semin Thorac Cardiovasc Surg 2007;19:206–11.

28. Eloubeidi MA, Cerfolio RJ, Chen VK, et al. Endoscopic ultrasound-guided fine needle aspiration of mediastinal lymph node in patients with suspected lung cancer after positron emission tomography and computed tomography scans. Ann Thorac Surg 2005;79:263–8.

29. Herth F, Beck R, Ernst A, et al. Conventional vs. endobronchial ultrasound-guided transbronchial needle aspiration: a randomized trial. Chest 2004;125:322–5.

30. Herth FJF, Eberhardt R, Becker HD, et al. Endobronchial ultrasound-guided transbronchial lung biopsy in fluoroscopically invisible solitary pulmonary nodules. A prospective trial. Chest 2006;129:147–50.

31. Yasufuku K, Nakajima T, Motoori K, et al. Comparison of endobronchial ultrasound, positron emission tomography, and CT for lymph node staging of lung cancer. Chest 2006;130:710–8.

32. Cerfolio RJ, Bryant AS, Eloubeidi MA, et al. Routine mediastinoscopy and esophageal ultrasound fine-needle aspiration in patients with non-small cell lung cancer who are clinically N2 negative: a prospective study. Chest 2006;130:1791–5.

33. Beamis JF. Interventional pulmonology techniques for treating malignant large airway obstruction: an update. Curr Opin Pulm Med 2005;11:292–5.

34. Asimakopoulos, Beeson J, Evans J, et al. Cryosurgery for malignant endobronchial tumors: analysis of outcome. Chest 2005;127:2007–14.

35. Chan AL, Yoneda KY, Allen RP, et al. Advances in the management of endobronchial lung malignancies. Curr Opin Pulm Med 2003;9:301–8.

36. Wood DE, Liu YH, Vallieres E, et al. Airway stenting for malignant and benign tracheobronchial stenosis. Ann Thorac Surg 2003;76:167–72.

37. Lee P, Kupeli E, Mehta AC, et al. Therapeutic bronchoscopy in lung cancer—laser therapy, electrocautery, brachytherapy stents, and photodynamic therapy. Clin Chest Med 2002;23:241.

38. Boiselle PM, Ernst A. State-of-the-art imaging of the central airways. Respiration 2003;70:383–94.

39. Lee KS, Lunn W, Feller-Kopman D, et al. Multislice CT evaluation of airway stents. J Thorac Imaging 2005;20:81–8.

40. Boiselle PM, FellerKopman D, Ashiku S, et al. Tracheobronchomalacia: evolving role of dynamic multislice helical CT. Radiol Clin North Am 2003;41:627.

41. Gluecker T, Lang F, Bessler S, et al. 2D and 3D CT imaging correlated to rigid endoscopy in complex laryngo-tracheal stenosis. Eur Radiol 2001;11:50–4.

42. Dialani V, Ernst A, Sun M, et al. MDCT detection of airway stent complications: comparison with bronchoscopy. AJR 2008;191:1576–80.

43. Ferretti GR, Kocier M, Calaque O, et al. Follow-up after stent insertion in the tracheobronchial tree: role of helical computed tomography in comparison with fiberoptic bronchoscopy. Eur Radiol 2003;13:1172–8.

44. Schreiber G, McCrory DC. Performance characteristics of different modalities for diagnosis of suspected lung cancer—summary of published evidence. Chest 2003;123:115S–28S.

45. Gaeta M, Pandolfo I, Volta S, et al. Bronchus sign on CT in peripheral carcinoma of the lung: value in predicting results of transbronchial biopsy. AJR Am J Roentgenol 1991;157:1181–5.

46. Naidich DP, Sussman R, Kutcher WL, et al. Solitary pulmonary nodules: CT-bronchoscopic correlation. Chest 1988;93:595–8.

47. Goldberg SN, Raptopoulos V, Boiselle PM, et al. Mediastinal lymph node biopsy: diagnostic yield of transbronchial mediastinal lymph node biopsy with CT fluoroscopic guidance—initial experience. Radiology 2000;216:764–7.

48. Asano F, Matsuno Y, Shinagawa N, et al. A virtual bronchoscopic navigation system for pulmonary peripheral lesions. Chest 2006;130:559–66.

49. Merritt SA, Gibbs JD, Yu K, et al. Image-guided bronchoscopy for peripheral lung lesions: a phantom study. Chest 2008;134:1017–26.

50. Shinagawa N, Yamazaki K, Onodera Y, et al. CT-guided transbronchial biopsy using an ultrathin bronchoscope with virtual bronchoscopic navigation. Chest 2004;125:1138–43.

51. Asahina H, Yamazaki K, Onodera Y, et al. Transbronchial biopsy using endobronchial ultrasonography with a guide sheath and virtual bronchoscopic navigation. Chest 2005;128:1761–4.

52. Sheski FD, Mathur PN. Endobronchial ultrasound. Chest 2008;133:264–70.

53. Paone G, Nicastri E, Lucantoni G, et al. Endobronchial ultrasound-driven biopsy in the diagnosis of peripheral lung lesions. Chest 2005;128:3551–7.

54. Schwarz Y, Grief J, Becker HD, et al. Real-time electromagnetic navigation bronchoscopy to peripheral lung lesions using overlaid CT images: the first human study. Chest 2006;129:988–94.

55. Schwarz Y, Mehta AC, Ernst A, et al. Electromagnetic navigation during flexible bronchoscopy. Respiration 2003;70:516–22.

56. Becker H, Herth F, Ernst A, et al. Bronchoscopic biopsy of peripheral lung lesion under electromagnetic guidance: a pilot study. J Bronchology 2005;12:9–13.

57. Eberhardt R, Anantham D, Herth F, et al. Electromagnetic navigation diagnostic bronchoscopy in peripheral lung lesions. Chest 2007;131:1800–5.

58. Gildea T, Mazzone P, Karnak D, et al. Electromagnetic navigation diagnostic bronchoscopy: a prospective study. Am J Respir Crit Care Med 2006;174:9982–9.

59. Makris D, Scherpereel A, Lerory S, et al. Electromagnetic navigation diagnostic bronchoscopy for small peripheral lung lesions. Eur Respir J 2007;29:1187–92.

60. Eberhardt R, Anantham D, Ernst A, et al. Multimodality bronchoscopic diagnosis of peripheral lung lesions. Am J Respir Crit Care Med 2007;176:36–41.

61. McLemore TL, Bedekar AR. Accurate diagnosis of peripheral lung lesions in a private community hospital employing electromagnetic guidance bronchoscopy (EMB) coupled with radial endobronchial ultrasound (REBUS). Chest 2007;132:452S.

62. Fishman A, Maartinez F, Naunheim K, et al. National Emphysema Treatment Trial research group. A randomized trial comparing lung-volume reduction surgery with medical therapy for severe emphysema. N Engl J Med 2003;348:2059–73.

63. Group. NETTR. Patients at high risk of death after lung-volume reduction surgery. N Engl J Med 2001;345:1075–83.

64. Brenner M, Hanna NM, Mina-Araghi R, et al. Innovative approaches to lung volume reduction for emphysema. Chest 2004;126:238–48.

65. Ingenito EP, Wood DE, Utz JP, et al. Bronchoscopic lung volume reduction in severe emphysema. Proc Am Thorac Soc 2008;5:454–60.

66. Sahi H, Karnak D, Meli YM, et al. Bronchoscopic approach to COPD. A review. COPD 2008;5:125–31.

67. Wood DE, McKenna RJ Jr, Yusen RD, et al. A multicenter trial of an intrabronchial valve for treatment of emphysema. J Thorac Cardiovasc Surg 2007;133:65–73.

68. Washko GR, Hoffman EA, Reilly JJ, et al. Radiographic evaluation of the potential lung volume reduction surgery candidate. Proc Am Thorac Soc 2008;5:421–6.

Bronchiectasis

Cylen Javidan-Nejad, MD*, Sanjeev Bhalla, MD

KEYWORDS

- Airway • Bronchiectasis • HRCT
- High-resolution CT • Cystic fibrosis • Ciliary dyskinesia

Bronchiectasis is defined as the irreversible dilatation of the cartilage-containing airways or bronchi. Enlargement of the bronchi in acute illness, as can be seen in the setting of infectious pneumonia, is usually reversible and would, therefore, not qualify as bronchiectasis (Fig. 1). Care must be taken to distinguish this large airway dilatation from dilatation of the small airways (bronchioles) that do not contain cartilage.[1]

MECHANISMS OF DEVELOPMENT

Bronchiectasis may result from one of three main mechanisms: bronchial wall injury, bronchial lumen obstruction, and traction from adjacent fibrosis.[2] The latter two mechanisms are usually apparent on imaging, and are suggested by an endobronchial filling defect or adjacent interstitial lung disease. It is when the first group is encountered that the radiologist is faced with a differential diagnosis and a potential diagnostic conondrum. In this article, we aim to cover the CT appearance of bronchiectasis, potential pitfalls, and a diagnostic approach to help narrow the diverse spectrum of conditions that may cause bronchiectasis.

Many conditions may lead to bronchial wall injury and subsequent bronchiectasis. These include infection and recurrent infections, impaired host defense leading to infection, exaggerated immune response, congenital structural defects of the bronchial wall, and extrinsic insults damaging the airway wall (Table 1). These conditions share the common denominator of mucus plugging and superimposed bacterial colonization. The mucus plugging is either a result of abnormal mucus constituency or abnormal mucus clearance. The toxins released by the bacteria and the cytokines and enzymes released by the surrounding inflammatory cells create

a vicious cycle of progressive wall damage, mucus plugging, and increased bacterial proliferation.[3,4] Once bronchiectasis begins, therefore, it is sure to progress.

Airway obstruction is most commonly caused by an intraluminal lesion such as carcinoid tumor, inflammatory myofibroblastic tumor, or a fibrous stricture usually from prior granulomatous infection such as histoplasmosis or tuberculosis. The presence of bronchiectasis can be useful in the differential diagnosis of an endoluminal mass, as its presence usually implies a chronic component. Although it may be seen with squamous cell carcinomas arising from papillomas, the presence of bronchiectasis is more suggestive of a slowly growing less malignant lesion, such as a carcinoid tumor (Fig. 2). Distal atelectasis and/or postobstructive pneumonitis are common in these conditions.[2] In the post lobectomy or post–lung transplant patient, granulation tissue at the suture line can occasionally result in an intraluminal occlusion and distal bronchiectasis. In these patients, immediate postoperative detection may allow for bronchoscopic removal of granulation tissue and avoid irreversible damage.

When bronchiectasis is from bronchial wall damage or bronchial obstruction, the bronchial wall becomes thickened because of infiltration by mononuclear cells and fibrosis. In cystic fibrosis (CF), an additional neutrophilic infiltration of the walls and airway lumen can be seen. This mural inflammatory process progressively destroys the elastin, muscle, and cartilage. This leads to airway dilatation.

The dilatation can be classified by its gross appearance as tubular (cylindric), varicose, or cystic (saccular). In the former, the bronchiectasis is manifest as parallel bronchial walls with failure of normal tapering and squared-off ends of the

Section of Cardiothoracic Imaging, Mallinckrodt Institute of Radiology, Washington University School of Medicine, 510 South Kingshighway, St. Louis, MO, USA
* Corresponding author.
E-mail address: javidanc@mir.wustl.edu (C. Javidan-Nejad).

Radiol Clin N Am 47 (2009) 289–306
doi:10.1016/j.rcl.2008.11.006
0033-8389/08/$ – see front matter. Published by Elsevier Inc.

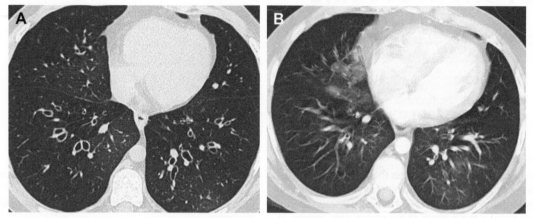

Fig. 1. Reversible lower lobe bronchial dilatation due to pneumonia. Initial CT (*A*) in this 12-year-old girl with hypogammaglobulinemia and pneumonia showed bilateral dilated lower lobe bronchi. Subsequent CT (*B*) performed 6 months later showed resolution of the bronchial dilatation, although it revealed a right middle lobe pneumonia. Because this dilatation is reversible, it would not qualify as bronchiectasis.

bronchus. As the process worsens, the bronchi become serpentine with a beaded appearance. This varicose bronchiectasis serves as an intermediate step before the development of grossly dilated, cystic airways. As the airway dilatation increases, there may be progressive collapse and fibrosis of the distal lung parenchyma.[2]

Traction bronchiectasis, as its name implies, is caused by retraction of mature fibrosis of the parenchyma around the bronchi. Such bronchiectasis follows the distribution of the underlying fibrosis. The traction bronchiectasis has an upper lobe distribution in cases of radiation fibrosis, sarcoidosis, and sequela of tuberculosis (Table 2) (Fig. 3). In cases of usual interstitial pneumonitis (UIP) (idiopathic pulmonary fibrosis) and fibrosing nonspecific interstitial pneumonitis (NSIP), the traction bronchiectasis tends to be mostly in the periphery and the lung bases (see Fig. 4).[5]

CLINICAL PRESENTATION AND DIAGNOSIS

Symptoms can be very nonspecific. Mild disease may manifest with a mild cough or minimal

Table 1
Bronchiectasis caused by airway wall damage

Mechanism	Disease
Congenital structural defect	Mounier-Kuhn syndrome
	William-Campbell syndrome
Infection	Pertussis (whooping cough)
	Tuberculosis
	Atypical mycobacterium
Impaired immune response	
Abnormal mucociliary clearance	Cystic fibrosis
	Primary ciliary dyskinesia
Decreased systemic immunity	Hypogammaglobulinemia
	Lung and bone transplantation
Exaggerated immune response	Allergic bronchopulmonary aspergillosis
	Inflammatory bowel disease
	c-ANCA-positive vasculitis
	Rheumatoid arthritis
Inhalational injury	Smoke and gaseous toxins
	Chronic gastroesophageal reflux and aspiration

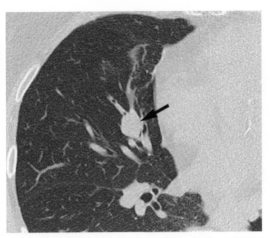

Fig. 2. Bronchiectasis due to obstructing carcinoid tumor. CT through the right middle lobe shows partially mucus-filled bronchiectasis and an endobronchial mass (*arrow*).

chronic hypoxemia and hypercarbia in more severe disease. Severe sinusitis can be seen if the bronchiectasis is due to primary cilia dyskinesia, Kartagener syndrome, cystic fibrosis, and diffuse panbronchiolitis.[6]

Hemoptysis, sometimes life-threatening, is caused by chronic airway inflammation and hypoxemia, which leads to bronchial arterial neovascularization.[7,8] These enlarged bronchial arteries are quite fragile and may rupture with even minimal trauma. Pulmonary hypertension can ensue because of underlying hypoxemic vasoconstriction and obstructive endarteritis.[9] The bronchial arteries anastamose with pulmonary arterioles, leading to left-to-right shunting, and if severe enough, can contribute to the pulmonary hypertension.[9]

The severity of airflow limitation is related to the extent and severity of the bronchiectasis. This can be seen in ventilation-perfusion mismatches and retained washout on the ventilation images of ventilation-perfusion scintigraphy. Decreased FEV1 (forced expiratory volume in 1 second) on spirometry can also be seen in the setting of bronchiectasis. Although useful in quantifying the ventilation impairment, spirometry has proven insensitive in detecting early structural damage.

dyspnea. As it becomes more severe, patients may present with chronic cough, regular and copious sputum production, progressive dyspnea, and repeated pulmonary infections.[3] Digital clubbing, anemia, and weight loss can develop because of

Table 2	
Bronchiectasis based on distribution	
Location	**Disease**
Focal	Congenital bronchial atresia
	Foreign body
	Broncholithiasis
	Endobronchial neoplasm
Diffuse	
Upper lung	Cystic fibrosis
	Sarcoidosis
	Progressive massive fibrosis of pneumoconiosis
	Radiation fibrosis
Central lung	Allergic bronchopulmonary aspergillosis
	End-stage hypersensitivity pneumonitis (also upper lobes)
	Mounier-Kuhn (also lower lobes if repeated infections)
Lower lung	Usual interstitial pneumonia (IPF)
	Nonspecific interstitial pneumonitis
	Hypogammaglobulinemia
	Lung and bone transplantation
	Chronic aspiration
	Idiopathic
Right middle lobe and lingula	Atypical mycobacterial infection
	Immotile cilia syndrome (PCD) (also lower lobes)

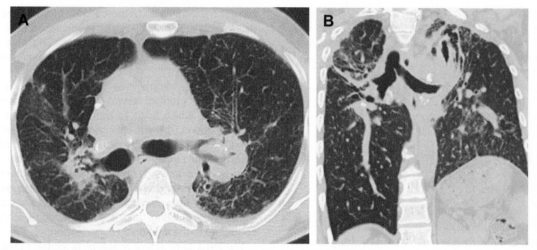

Fig. 3. Upper lobe traction bronchiectasis from end-stage sarcoid. Transaxial image at the level of the carina (A) demonstrates tortuous, shortened bronchi amidst upper lobe fibrosis and volume loss. Upper lobe predominance of the bronchiectasis is better appreciated on coronal reconstruction (B).

Because of the insensitivity of the other techniques and the high-spatial resolution of CT, high-resolution computed tomography (HRCT) has become the favored diagnostic tool for detection of bronchiectasis.[10,11] Rapid disease progression has a poorer prognosis and has been shown to be associated with increased wall thickening, colonization by *Pseudomonas aeruginosa*, and high concentrations of proinflammatory markers in sputum or serum, such as neutrophilic elastase.[4,12]

Diagnosis is usually suspected by history and confirmed by spirometry and HRCT. Depending on the associated symptoms and age of presentation, the diagnostic workup may include a sweat electrolyte test, serum immunoglobulin levels, or serum *Aspergillus* antibody and precipitin, or even genetic testing. Occasionally electron microscopy of the ciliated cells may be used.[6]

Bronchoscopy is diagnostic and sometimes therapeutic. In localized bronchiectasis caused by a foreign body, an endobronchial neoplasm, bronchiolithiasis, and fibrotic stenosis, bronchoscopy may be used to remove the obstructing lesion. Although the bronchiectasis itself will not revert, the clearance of the airway will improve any postobstructive pneumonia and may prevent progression of the airway damage.[13] Bronchoscopy and lavage is helpful in patients with more diffuse bronchiectasis who present with acute

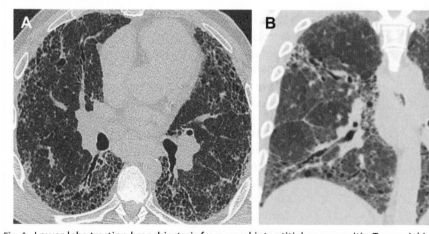

Fig. 4. Lower lobe traction bronchiectasis from usual interstitial pneumonitis. Transaxial image at the level of the superior segmental bronchi (A) demonstrates traction bronchiectasis, within peripheral-dominant honeycombing in this 52-year-old man with idiopathic pulmonary fibrosis. Coronal reformatted image (B) shows that the basilar and peripheral bronchiectasis follows the distribution of the fibrosis.

exacerbation or sudden worsening of underlying symptoms. This is usually a sign of acute airway infection, commonly by *Pseudomonas* and *Staphylococcus*, and in such patients bronchoscopy is helpful in obtaining samples for culture and determining antibiotic sensitivity, when usual measures of sputum sampling are unsuccessful.[6]

HIGH-RESOLUTION CT IMAGING TECHNIQUE

Because of the nonspecific nature of symptoms associated with bronchiectasis, an accurate way of diagnosis is needed. HRCT provides the most accurate, least invasive technique. It enables the assessment of bronchial abnormalities to the level of the secondary pulmonary lobule level. Conventional HRCT is performed by acquiring 1.0- to 1.5-mm thick images, every 10 mm, reconstructed using a high spatial frequency algorithm. Images can be obtained in a spiral or sequential mode. Using conventional technique, visualization of bronchi 1 to 2 mm in diameter and vessels 0.1 to 0.2 mm in diameter may be achieved.[1] The lungs are scanned twice, during suspended end- inhalation and suspended end-exhalation. The latter phase is performed to reveal subtle air trapping.

Multidetector computed tomography (MDCT) scanners allow fast, volumetric data acquisition, creating contiguous thin sections through the lungs with excellent z-axis spatial resolution. Similar scanning technique is used for all multidetector scanners that have 16 detector rows or higher, where a collimation of 0.50 to 1.25 mm is selected. The scans are performed in inspiration and reconstructed as contiguous 1-mm images or 1-mm-thick images with 10-mm reconstruction interval. Additional advantages are improved anatomic matching of airways with regions of air trapping during inspiration and expiration and providing the ability for postprocessing the axial images to create 3-dimensional (3D) assessment of the airways.[14,15] These postprocessed multiplanar images have become known as volumetric HRCT.[16]

In our center, we use a 16- or 64-row multidetector scanner and image the thorax without use of intravenous contrast during end-inspiration and end-exhalation. Inspiration images are acquired helically and reconstructed as 5×5-mm images and 1×10-mm images; 1×1-mm images are also created in case any mutiplanar or 3D imaging is needed. Exhalation images are also obtained helically and reconstructed as 1×10 mm.

When radiation dose is a consideration (especially in younger patients), a low-dose technique of 30 mAs is used in the expiratory phase. A growing number of authors have advocated the use of low-dose techniques for HRCT, but we have not routinely relied on these.[17]

IMAGING FINDINGS

The imaging findings on conventional radiography are based on visualizing the bronchial wall thickening. This results in ill-defined perihilar linear densities associated with indistinctness of the margins of the central pulmonary arteries. This appearance simulates interstitial pulmonary edema, but lacks the peripheral Kerley B lines. When the bronchus is seen on end, ill-defined ring shadows can be identified because of bronchial wall thickening. The presence of tram lines or parallel lines along the expected courses of the bronchi indicates more severe bronchiectasis, where the dilated bronchial lumen becomes visible on conventional radiography. Tram lines are best identified in the lower lobes, right middle lobe, and lingula (**Fig. 5**). Oftentimes, an abnormality is detected but the specific diagnosis of bronchiectasis is not.

Mucus plugging may appear as elongated opacities, which may be sometimes calcified. These tubular opacities can be confused for pulmonary vascular enlargement. In cystic bronchiectasis, air-fluid levels in thick-walled cysts are seen, associated with variable degrees of surrounding consolidations and atelectasis. Based on the cause and extent of bronchiectasis, the overall lung volume may be increased (**Fig. 6**).[1,2,6]

CT, especially HRCT, is quite reliable in diagnosing bronchiectasis. On CT a diagnosis of bronchiectasis is made when the internal luminal diameter of one or more bronchi exceeds the diameter of the adjacent artery. Other diagnostic criteria of bronchiectasis are the lack of normal tapering of a bronchus, a visible bronchus abutting the mediastinal pleura, or a visible bronchus within 1 cm of the pleura. Signs of bronchiectasis on CT include the signet ring sign, denoted by the artery simulating a jewel abutting the ring, the thick-walled dilated bronchus on a transaxial view, and the tram-track sign, from parallel, thickened walls of a dilated bronchus (**Fig. 7**).

In cylindric bronchiectasis the luminal dilatation is uniform and the wall thickening is smooth. Varicose bronchiectasis denotes a more severe form of disease, where the luminal dilatation is characterized by alternating areas of luminal dilatation and constriction, creating a beaded appearance, and the wall thickening is irregular. In cystic bronchiectasis, the most severe form of bronchiectasis, a dilated, thick-walled bronchus terminates in a thick-walled cyst.[18] Oftentimes, more than

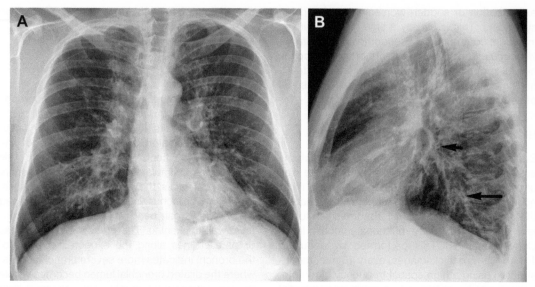

Fig. 5. Diffuse bronchiectasis on conventional radiography. Diffuse bronchiectasis can obscure the perihilar vascular markings, similar to early interstitial pulmonary edema on a pulmonary artery (PA) radiograph (*A*). Identifying dilated bronchi on end (*short arrow*) and tram lines (*long arrow*) leads to the correct diagnosis of bronchiectasis. In this case of cystic fibrosis in a 42-year-old man, the findings are best seen on the lateral radiograph (*B*).

one type of bronchiectasis can be seen in the same patient (**Fig. 8**).

Smooth bronchial wall thickening is seen in all cases of bronchiectasis, except those caused by congenital cartilage deficiency (William-Campbell syndrome, Mounier-Kuhn syndrome) or in allergic bronchopulmonary aspergillosis (ABPA). Bronchial wall thickening alone is a nonspecific finding, as it is also seen in asthma and chronic bronchitis.[6]

A potential pitfall in the diagnosis of bronchiectasis is the double image of a vessel created by cardiac or respiratory motion artifact simulating a dilated bronchus. This is most common in the lingula and left lower lobe where the effect of cardiac motion is most prominent (**Fig. 9**). Caution should be made when diagnosis of bronchial wall thickening is made on HRCT images that have been reconstructed with a very high frequency algorithm.

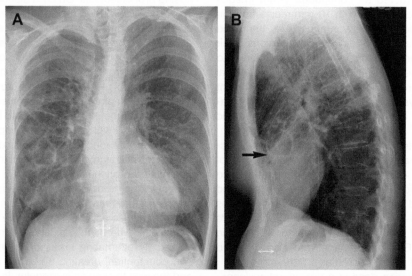

Fig. 6. Cystic bronchiectasis on conventional radiography. Cystic changes are seen in both mid and lower lungs (*arrows*) on the PA chest radiograph (*A*) in this 61-year-old woman with chronic *Mycobacterium avium* intracellulare/complex (MAC) infection. The lateral (*B*) radiograph demonstrates an air-fluid level in cystic bronchiectasis of the right middle lobe (*arrow*).

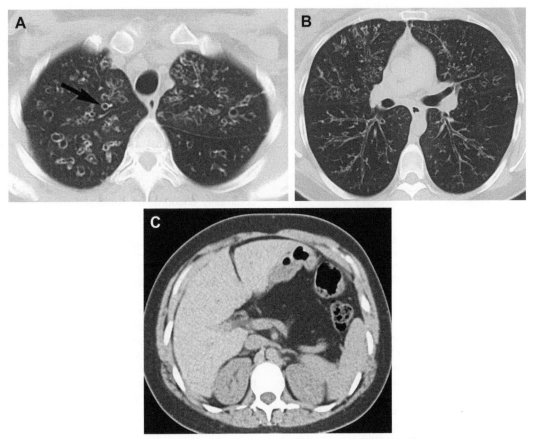

Fig. 7. CT findings of diffuse bronchiectasis in a 27-year-old woman with cystic fibrosis. Transaxial images show the dilated bronchus and adjacent arteriole, seen along their short axis, creating the signet ring sign (*arrow*) (*A*). When the bronchi are visualized along their course, the lack of normal tapering and smooth bronchial wall thickening can be appreciated (*B*). In cystic fibrosis the fatty attenuation of the pancreas is indicative of the pancreatic insufficiency (*C*).

Such algorithm causes the interstitium to appear very thickened and the prominence of the bronchial walls results in a "pseudo-bronchiectasis" appearance (**Fig. 10**).

Mucus plugging of the dilated bronchi and bronchioles appear as branching dense tubular structures, coursing parallel to, but thicker in diameter, than the adjacent artery and arteriole. These

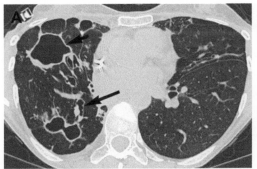
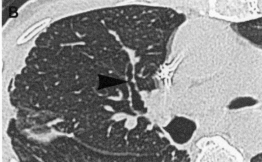

Fig. 8. CT findings of varicose and cystic bronchiectasis. CT images from the same patient as in Fig. 6 show a more severe form of bronchiectasis, where both varicose (*long arrow*) and cystic (*short arrow*) bronchiectasis is present (*A*). In varicose bronchiectasis, the bronchial lumen has a beaded appearance and nodular wall thickening is seen (*arrowhead*) (*B*).

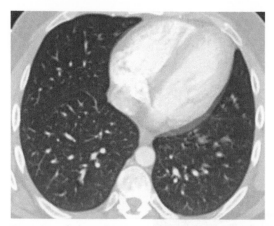

Fig. 9. Pseudo-bronchiectasis due to cardiac motion. The cardiac motion creates a double image, simulating bronchiectasis, usually seen in the left lower lobe and lingula. The artifactual nature of this observation is confirmed by the motion artifact along the posterior wall of the heart.

plugged bronchi are accompanied by adjacent aggregates of nodules, in a "tree-in-bud" pattern, consistent with mucus-filled bronchiolectasis in the center of the secondary pulmonary lobule (**Fig. 11**).

Mosaic attenuation and air trapping are common associated findings. This is felt to be because of coexisting constrictive bronchiolitis in patients with bronchiectasis. The air trapping may be more pronounced when the bronchiectatic airway has a component of bronchomalacia (**Fig. 12**).

BRONCHIECTASIS BASED ON ETIOLOGY

A majority of bronchiectasis encountered in clinical practice will be postinfectious in origin. In fact, in two retrospective studies evaluating the etiology of bronchiectasis in large cohorts of patients with bronchiectasis, almost one third of the patients were found to have bronchiectasis from prior infection. Idiopathic bronchiectasis, where despite extensive workup the cause was not found, and bronchiectasis related to abnormal mucociliary clearance (cystic fibrosis and primary ciliary dyskinesia) each accounted for almost a quarter of the cases. ABPA and systemic immunodeficiency, due to congenital and acquired causes, were the next most common causes.[3,19] Some of the more commonly encountered etiologies are presented in the following sections.

Traction Bronchiectasis

Traction bronchiectasis is common in UIP, NSIP, and sarcoid and end-stage hypersensitivity pneumonitis.[20,21]

The mechanism of bronchiectasis in fibrotic lung is based on both physiology and mechanical forces involved in inspiration. Patients with widespread fibrosis require increased inspiratory work, leading to a more negative pleural pressure and therefore a greater transpulmonary pressure during inspiration. On the other hand, pulmonary fibrosis increases the elastic recoil of the lung, creating even further expansion of the bronchi during inspiration.

In our practice, we find it helpful to compare bronchiectasis to the adjacent fibrosis. When the bronchiectasis is out of proportion with the adjacent fibrosis, then NSIP secondary to collagen vascular disease may be considered. The explanation may stem from bronchial wall injury caused by collagen vascular disease–related inflammation or secondary to the high incidence of chronic aspiration in this subgroup of patients (**Fig. 13**).

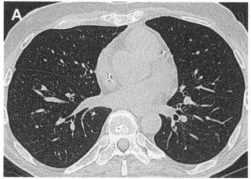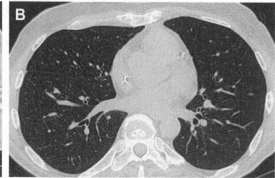

Fig. 10. Imaging pitfall. A very sharp reconstruction algorithm (B80f) of the CT image may result in increased noise, creating the illusion of bronchial wall thickening (*A*). When the same image is reconstructed with a less sharp algorithm (B60f), it becomes clear that the bronchiectasis is not real (*B*).

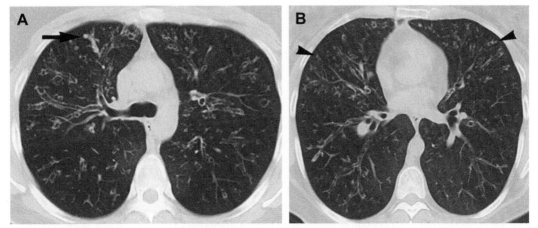

Fig. 11. Mucus plugging on CT. On transaxial images, the filling of bronchiectasis by mucus appears as tubular and branching opacities, with club-like, rounded ends (*arrow*) (*A*). The mucus-filled smaller branching bronchi and bronchioles appear as tree-in-bud opacities (*arrowheads*) (*B*). The mosaic attenuation of the surrounding lung is due to air trapping. In this case, the bronchiectasis was from cystic fibrosis.

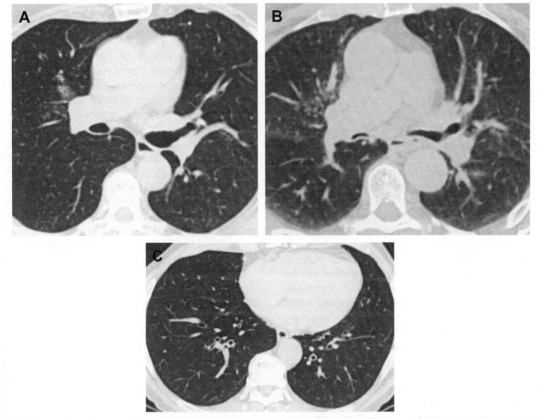

Fig. 12. Bronchomalacia and bronchiectasis: a 68-year-old man with a reported history of asthma nonresponsive to steroid therapy. CT images show a normal caliber of the central bronchi (*A*), and marked collapse of their lumina when imaged during forced exhalation (*B*), consistent with bronchomalacia. The distal bronchi are diffusely dilated and have smooth wall thickening, consistent with mild bronchiectasis (*C*).

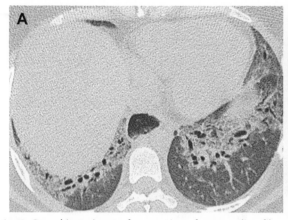 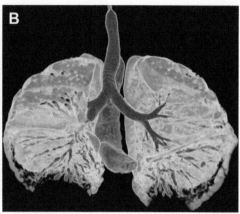

Fig. 13. Bronchiectasis out of proportion of surrounding fibrosis. Transaxial CT of the chest of a 34-year-old woman with scleroderma shows a dilated esophagus, basilar pulmonary fibrosis, and significant bronchiectasis without evidence of honeycombing (*A*). The volume-rendered image demonstrates the extent of the bronchiectasis (*B*) and the markedly dilated esophagus.

Congenital Airway Wall Abnormality

Congenital defects of the cartilage, collagen, or other components of the bronchial wall lead to abnormal physiologic clearing of mucoid excretions, predisposing the bronchial epithelium to repeated infections and a vicious cycle of progressive bronchial dilatation. Structural wall defect is the common feature of Mounier-Kuhn disease or tracheobronchomegaly, William-Campbell syndrome, and congenital bronchial atresia.

TRACHEOBRONCHOMEGALY (MOUNIER-KUHN DISEASE)

Tracheobronchomegaly is an uncommon disease that presents mostly in men, in the fourth and fifth decades. Although believed to be congenital, it may be associated with Ehlers-Danlos syndrome, Marfan syndrome, and generalized elastosis (cutis laxa). Pathological thinning of the muscle, cartilage, and elastic tissue of the airway walls is seen. This results in uniform dilatation of the tracheal and bronchial lumina and increased distensibility of the tracheal and bronchial walls. This tracheobronchomalacia leads to recurrent infections in the dependent lungs.[6]

The disease involves the entire trachea and bronchi of first to fourth order. On imaging, a tracheal diameter exceeding 3 cm in both coronal and sagittal planes and central bronchiectasis is seen without associated airway wall thickening. More distal bronchiectasis, bronchial wall thickening, occasionally fibrosis, and cystic changes in the lower lobes are common because of sequela of repeated pneumonia.[22,23] The net effect is

a progression of the bronchiectasis and lung disease, which, in turn, may result in increased tracheobronchomegaly (**Fig. 14**).

CONGENITAL BRONCHIAL ATRESIA OR MUCOCELE

A focal area of bronchiectasis surrounded by lucent lung is typical of congenital bronchial atresia or congenital mucocele. This condition is characterized by congenital focal obliteration of the lumen of a segmental bronchus, resulting in focal bronchiectasis and air trapping more distally. The dilated airway is commonly filled by inspissated mucus, which may occasionally calcify. Congenital bronchial atresia is usually focal, and is commonly discovered incidentally, as an ovoid, tubular, or branching density on a chest radiograph. It may be confused with a pulmonary nodule. CT reveals its bronchial, branching nature, and the presence of surrounding and more distal hyperexpanded and hyperlucent lung parenchyma, due to the associated air trapping (**Fig. 15**).

Conversely, acquired mucocele is caused by focal scarring of a segmental bronchus because of prior granulomatous infection or from an endobronchial lesion. It should be differentiated from congenital bronchial atresia by the absence of air trapping of the distal lung parenchyma.[24,25] The presence of an acquired mucocele should prompt further interrogation to exclude the possibility of an endobronchial neoplasm (**Fig. 16**).

WILLIAMS-CAMPBELL SYNDROME

Williams-Campbell syndrome is a rare disease in which the cartilage of the fourth-, fifth-, and

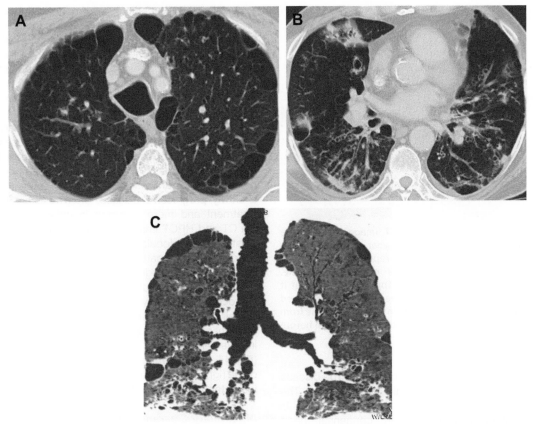

Fig. 14. Mounier-Kuhn Syndrome. Transaxial CT images show tracheomegaly (*A*), and basilar-predominant varicose and cystic bronchiectasis (*B*) seen in Mounier-Kuhn syndrome. The coronal reconstructed image demonstrates the typical corrugated appearance of the tracheal wall (*C*).

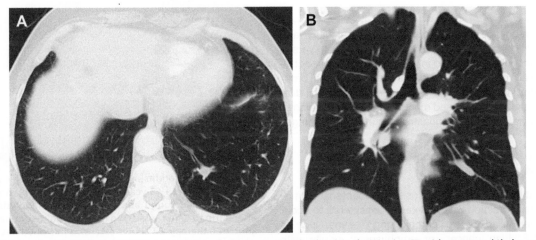

Fig. 15. Congenital bronchial atresia: a 60-year-old woman with pleuritic chest pain. CT with contrast (*A*) shows a nodular density in the left lower lobe with surrounding hyperlucency of the lung parenchyma, due to focal air trapping. Coronal reconstruction (*B*) better demonstrates the tubular nature of that structure, which connects to a dilated bronchus. These features (mucocele with surrounding air trapping) are diagnostic for this condition.

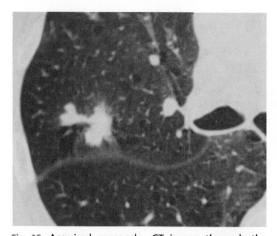

Fig. 16. Acquired mucocele. CT image through the right upper lobe in this 68-year-old man reveals a branching tubular structure representing a mucus-filed dilated subsegmental bronchus or mucocele. The lack of surrounding air trapping suggests that it is not congenital and likely because of an acquired obstruction of the bronchus. In this case, it was from a small squamous cell cancer that was not seen before surgery.

sixth-generation bronchi is defective. The disease may involve the lung focally or diffusely.[26] The congenital form presents in childhood and is commonly associated with congenital heart disease, polysplenia, bronchial isomerism, and situs inversus. The acquired form is likely a sequela of prior adenovirus (measles and pertussis) infections.[27] CT imaging shows cystic bronchiectasis distal to the third-generation bronchi, and inspiratory-expiratory CT imaging reveals ballooning on inspiration and collapse on exhalation.[1]

Acquired Wall Abnormalities

Chronic or past infections, inhalational injury, and cellular infiltration in the setting of graft versus host disease lead to inflammation of the bronchial wall, resulting in structural damage of the bronchial wall. This leads to irreversible bronchial dilatation and increased mucus production, leading to a vicious cycle of inflammation and wall damage.

ATYPICAL OR NONTUBERCULOSIS MYCOBACTERIA

Atypical or nontuberculosis mycobacterial pulmonary infection was previously considered to occur only in adults with chronic lung disease, such as CF, lung cancer, or emphysema; adults with impaired immunity, especially acquired immunodeficiency syndrome (AIDS), or those with thoracic skeletal abnormalities. These organisms, however,

especially mycobacterium avium intracellulare-complex (MAC), are increasingly being recognized as the cause of chronic lung infection in adults with normal immunity and no underlying lung disease, especially older women. In immunocompetent people, MAC has three different forms: a fibrocavitary form, a nodular bronchiectatic form, and hypersensitivity pneumonitis.

The fibrocavitary form, similar to postprimary tuberculosis, involves the apices and upper lobes and causes traction bronchiectasis in the affected lung. It occurs mostly in older men with emphysema. The nodular bronchiectasis form represents a slowly progressive disease, often resistant to treatment and more common in older women. On CT and HRCT imaging it appears as multiple clusters of centrilobular micronodules, in a branching or tree-in-bud pattern, aggregating around air- or mucus-filled cylindric bronchiectasis and bronchiolectasis. Multifocal consolidations and cavities can occur. There is associated mosaic attenuation and air trapping. The disease has a predilection for the right middle lobe, upper lobes, and lingula, but involvement of other lobes may also be seen (Fig. 17).[28–30] Scarring and traction bronchiectasis of the right middle lobe and lingula are indicative of long-standing disease (Fig. 18).

Mucociliary Clearance Abnormalities

The ciliary ladder is responsible for effective clearing of mucoid excretions of the airway epithelium. Abnormalities in the consistency of mucus in

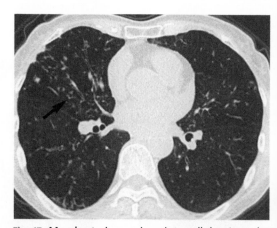

Fig. 17. Mycobacterium avium intracellulare/complex (MAC) infection: a 68-year-old Chinese woman who developed mild cough and intermittent hemoptysis after a trip to China, which did not respond to routine antibiotic therapy. CT shows extensive micronodules, mostly in the right middle lobe, right lower lobe, and lingula, which aggregate in a tree-in-bud pattern around the mildly dilated subsegmental bronchi (*arrow*). Sputum specimen was positive for MAC.

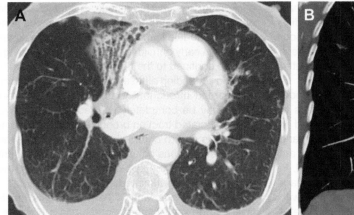
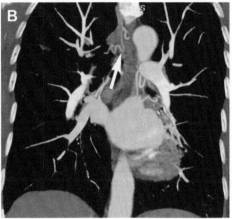

Fig. 18. Bronchial artery collateral formation in bronchiectasis: a 76-year-old woman with chronic productive cough has new-onset of severe, recurrent hemoptysis. CT of chest with intravenous contrast shows severe bronchiectasis and scarring of the right middle lobe (A). The dilated bronchial arteries (*white arrow*) providing collateral flow to the lungs are better demonstrated on the coronal thin-MIP (6 mm) reformatted image (B).

cystic fibrosis, and abnormalities of the structure and function of the cilia of the airway epithelium, as seen in primary ciliary dyskinesia or immotile ciliary syndrome, leads to ineffective mucus clearance and secondary colonization of the airway lumina by bacteria. This chronic infection and repeated bouts of pneumonia lead to bronchiectasis. The bronchiectasis of cystic fibrosis is typically worse in the upper lobes, as opposed to primary and acquired ciliary dyskinesia, such as Young syndrome where bronchiectasis is associated with azospermia, where the bronchiectasis is worse in the dependant or lower lungs.

CYSTIC FIBROSIS

CF is an autosomal recessive trait and occurs in approximately 1 in 3000 live births in the United States and Europe. It is caused by a mutation in the CF transmembrane conductance regulator (CFTR). This results in failed secretion of chloride through the CFTR and associated ion channels, leading to dehydration of the endobronchial secretions. This thickened mucus cannot be efficiently cleared by the mucociliary system, leading to obstructed airways and bacterial infection.[4] Colonization and recurrent infection with

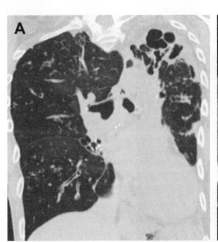
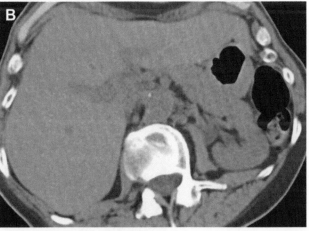

Fig. 19. Initial diagnosis of cystic fibrosis late in life. A 68-year-old woman had undergone left lower lobectomy more than 35 years ago because of recurrent pneumonia of the left lower lobe. Recent dyspnea on exertion and wheezing prompted further workup, which revealed a sweat chloride = 81 mmol/L (normal <40 mmol/L). Coronal reformatted image of HRCT of chest (A) shows severe bronchiectasis of the left upper lobe, and relatively mild bronchiectasis throughout the right lung. Transaxial nonenhanced CT of abdomen does not show fatty pancreatic parenchyma (B).

Staphylococcus aureus, Haemophilus influenza, and *Pseudomonas aeruginosa* is common, leading to progression of airway destruction. A poor prognosis is made when atypical mycobacteria or *Burkholderia cepacia* colonize the dilated airways.[6]

Although CF is usually diagnosed in childhood, the heterogeneity of severity of disease leads to patients with milder disease, first diagnosed in adulthood. As genetic testing improves and awareness of CF increases, milder forms are increasingly being detected later in adulthood. In fact, at our institution, the oldest first-time diagnosis of CF was in a 72-year-old woman with mild bronchiectasis. Sweat chloride test greater than 40 mmol/L indicates the presence of disease.

CT findings include diffuse cylindric, varicose, or even cystic bronchiectasis, bronchial wall thickening. Extensive mucus plugging of the dilated bronchi and bronchioles manifests as centrilobular nodules and branching densities (see **Fig. 7**).[1] In early or mild forms of CF, these findings may be confined to the right upper lobe.[6] In adults with long-standing diffuse disease, the findings are widespread throughout the lungs and the upper lobes may be completely scarred and collapsed with associated traction bronchiectasis. This lobar scarring is due to chronicity of disease where the bronchiectasis has been most severe and present longest. Despite the upper lobe volume loss, the lungs remain hyperinflated.

Typically patients with CF have pancreatic insufficiency and on CT the pancreas has a homogenous fat attenuation. However, in cases of a milder mutation, which leads to an initial diagnosis later in life, the pancreatic insufficiency is commonly absent (**Fig. 19**).[31]

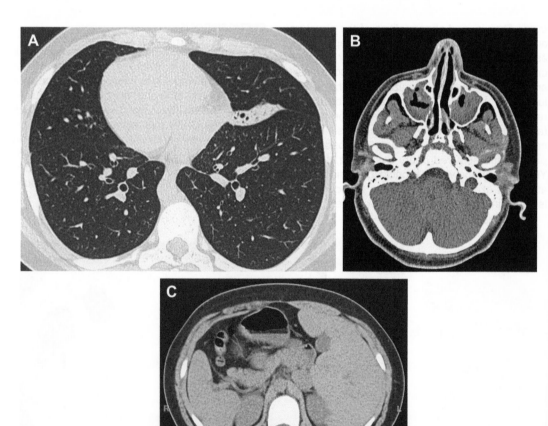

Fig. 20. Kartagener syndrome. Transaxial CT of chest (*A*) in a 12-year-old boy with Kartagener Syndrome shows dextrocardia and bronchiectasis of the lower lobes and scarring of the left middle lobe caused by more severe bronchiectasis and repeated pneumonia. Nonenhanced CT of the paranasal sinuses (*B*) show marked mucosal thickening and opacification of the maxillary sinuses. The transaxial nonenhanced CT image of the upper abdomen (*C*) demonstrates the situs inversus associated with this syndrome.

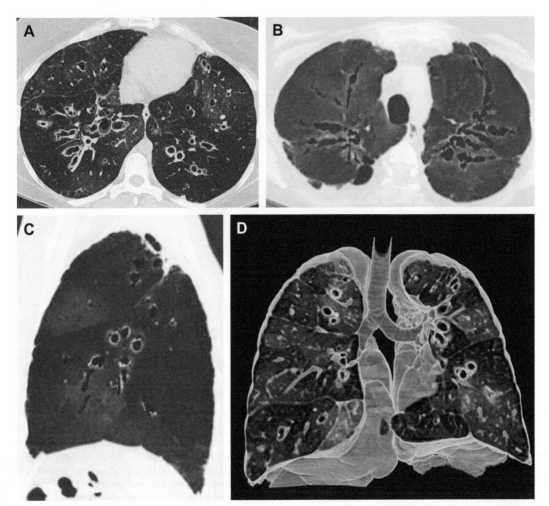

Fig. 21. Primary ciliary dyskinesia: a 37-year-old woman with primary ciliary dyskinesia and chronic pseudomonas aeruginosa infection being evaluated for bilateral lung transplantation. HRCT of chest (A) shows mixed tubular, varicose, and cystic bronchiectasis. Minimal intensity reformatted images in axial (B) and sagittal (C) planes and volume-rendered image (D) demonstrate the extent of bronchiectasis and the associated mosaic attenuation.

PRIMARY CILIARY DYSKINESIA

Primary ciliary dyskinesia (PCD) or immotile ciliary syndrome is caused by a defect in structure and function of the airway cilia. This leads to impaired mucociliary clearance.[32] It is a genetically heterogeneous, autosomal recessive trait with a prevalence of approximately 1 in 15,000 to 1 in 30,000 of live births. Patients present with recurrent infections of the lungs, sinuses, and middle ear. Similar to CF, PCD causes progressive bronchiectasis. Thoracoabdominal asymmetry occurs in approximately 50% of patients. Kartagener syndrome or triad is present in half of the PCD patients. This triad consists of situs inversus, bronchiectasis, and sinusitis (Fig. 20).[33,34]

PCD tends to be diagnosed relatively late, because of its nonspecific presenting symptoms in children. Clinical suspicion based on a focused history leads to diagnosis. The current diagnostic test of choice is electron microscopic analysis of respiratory cilia in samples of nasal or airway mucosa. This reveals defects in the outer or inner dynein arms of the cilia.[33]

The CT findings of PCD are bronchiectasis of variable severity, associated with tree-in-bud nodules and branching densities because of mucus plugging, and lobar scarring and air trapping (Fig. 21). Bronchiectasis in PCD is predominantly in the lingual and middle and lower lobes of the lung. Isolated upper lobe involvement and isolated peripheral bronchiectasis is very rare.

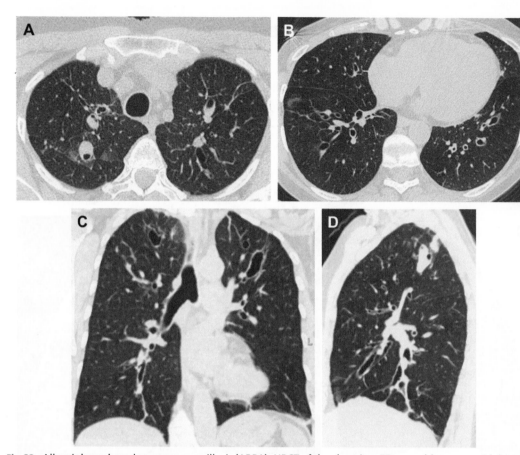

Fig. 22. Allergic bronchopulmonary aspergillosis (ABPA). HRCT of the chest in a 55-year-old woman with history of reactive airway disease at the level of the apices (*A*) and lung bases (*B*) show dilated, thick-walled bronchi. The bronchiectasis is worse in the apices where mucus plugging is seen. Coronal (*C*) and sagittal (*D*) reformatted images better demonstrate the distribution of the bronchiectasis.

Hyper-Immune Response

Inflammatory bowel disease, rheumatoid arthritis, Sjogren disease, antineutrophilic cytoplasmic antibody (c-ANCA)–positive vasculitis (Wegener disease), and allergic bronchopulmonary aspergillosis all can lead to bronchiectasis, possibly because of inflammation of the airway wall in the setting of a hyperimmune response to internal or external antigens. The chronic inflammation damages the bronchial walls, leading to bronchiectasis.

ALLERGIC BRONCHOPULMONARY ASPERGILLOSIS

Allergic brochopulmonary aspergillosis (ABPA) is due to a hypersensitivity reaction to *Aspergillus fumigatis* antigens, leading to development of bronchocentric granulomata in the bronchi and bronchioles, associated with mucus impaction.[35] It is most commonly seen in patients with atopic rhinitis, asthma, or CF.[36] Patients present with wheezing, fever, and pleuritic chest pain and

may cough up brown mucus plugs. Clinical diagnosis could be made by detecting an elevated serum IgE level, eosinophilia on peripheral blood smears, or positive skin reaction to *Aspergillus* antigen. Mycelia can occasionally be identified in the exporated mucus plugs.

Chest radiographs and CT show migratory pneumonitis early in the disease. This usually involves the upper lobes. Central and upper lobe bronchiectasis, varicose or cystic subtypes, is best detected by CT, which also helps monitor progression and response to treatment. In more chronic disease, inspissated mucus in the dilated central bronchi created the appearance of the classic finger-in-glove appearance on the chest radiographs (**Fig. 22**). Atelectasis or hyperinflation of the lung distal to the impacted bronchi can occur.[18,35]

SUMMARY

Bronchiectasis, or the irreversible dilatation of bronchi, can present with a host of nonspecific clinical symptoms, including hemoptysis, cough, and hypoxia. The radiologist, then, can play an important role in its detection and characterization. Bronchiectasis must be differentiated from motion artifact and transient bronchial dilatation in acute lung disease. When diagnosed, a logical approach may allow for proper triage of the patient to prevent progression of disease.

The radiologic approach usually begins with CT, which is fast and accurate. The diagnostic approach should be based on the mechanisms of development of bronchiectasis (bronchial wall damage, endobronchial obstruction, and traction) and the location. Once an endobronchial lesion or adjacent fibrosis is excluded, location of the abnormality can be used to help narrow the differential diagnosis. When the bronchiectasis is upper lobe predominant, CF should first be considered but occasionally MAC infection may present with this finding. When the bronchiectasis is mid-upper lobe, then ABPA or chronic hypersensitivity pneumonitis might lead the list of diagnoses. Lower lobe bronchiectasis is usually the sequela of recurrent infection and conditions that predispose to recurrent infections, including Mounier-Kuhn, hypogammaglobulinemia, PCD, and recurrent infections. By using this approach, the radiologist can remain an integral part of the pulmonary team.

REFERENCES

1. Hartman TE, Primack SL, Lee KS, et al. CT of bronchial and bronchiolar diseases. Radiographics 1994;14:991–1003.

2. Shoemark A, Ozerovitch L, Wilson R. Aetiology in adult patients with bronchiectasis. Respir Med 2007;191:1163–70.

3. Muller NL, Fraser RS, Lee KS, et al. Diseases of the lung—radiologic and pathologic correlations. 1st edition. [chapter 15]. Philadelphia: Lippincott Williams and Wilkins; 2003. p. 280–1.

4. Lynch DA, Newell JD, Lee JS. Imaging of diffuse lung disease. 1st edition. [chapter 6]. Hamilton (ON): B.C.Decker Inc; 2000. p. 175–86.

5. Westcott JL, Cole SR. Traction bronchiectasis in end-stage pulmonary fibrosis. Radiology 1986;161: 665–9.

6. Hirshberg B, Biran I, Glazer M, et al. Hemoptysis: etiology, evaluation, and outcome in a tertiary referral hospital. Chest 1997;112:440–4.

7. Bruzzi JF, Remy-Jardin M, Delhaye D, et al. Multidetector row CT of hemoptysis. Radiographics 2006; 26:3–22.

8. Alzeer AH, Al-Mobeirek AF, Al-Otair HAK, et al. Right and left ventricular function and pulmonary artery pressure in patients with bronchiectasis. Chest 2008;133:468–73.

9. Chang AB, Masel JP, Boyce MC, et al. Non-CF bronchiectasis: clinical and HRCT evaluation. Pediatr Pulmonol 2003;35:477–83.

10. Eshed I, Minski I, Katz R, et al. Bronchiectasis: correlation of high-resolution CT findings with health-related quality of life. Clin Radiol 2007;62: 152–9.

11. Martınez-Garcıa MA, Soler-Cataluna JJ, Perpina-Tordera M, et al. Factors associated with lung function decline in adult patients with stable non-cystic fibrosis bronchiectasis. Chest 2007;132: 1565–72.

12. Camacho JR, Prakash UB. 46 year old man with chronic hemoptysis. Mayo Clin Proc 1995;70:83–6.

13. Kwong JS, Muller NL, Miller RR. Diseases of the trachea and main-stem bronchi: correlation of CT with pathologic findings. Radiographics 1992;12: 645–57.

14. Di Scioscio V, Zompatori M, Mistura I, et al. The role of spiral multidetector dynamic CT in the study of Williams-Campbell syndrome. Acta Radiol 2006; 47(8):798–800.

15. Carden KA, Boiselle PM, Waltz DA, et al. Tracheomalacia and tracheobronchomalacia in children and adults: an in-depth review. Chest 2005;127: 984–1005.

16. Nishino M, Hatabu H. Volumetric expiratory HRCT imaging with MSCT. J Thorac Imaging 2005;20(3): 176–85.

17. de Jong PA, Nakano Y, Lequin MH, et al. Dose reduction for CT in children with cystic fibrosis: is it feasible to reduce the number of images per scan? Pediatr Radiol 2006;36(1):50–3.

18. Elizur A, Cannon CL, Ferkol TW. Airway inflammation in cystic fibrosis. Chest 2008;133:489–95.

19. Robinson TE. Computed tomography scanning techniques for the evaluation of cystic fibrosis lung disease. Proc Am Thorac Soc 2007;4:310–5.

20. Kennedy MP, Noone PG, Leigh MW, et al. High-resolution CT of patients with primary ciliary dyskinesia. AJR Am J Roentgenol 2007;188:1232–8.

21. Pasteur MC, Helliwell SM, Houghton SJ, et al. An investigation into causative factors in patients with bronchiectasis. Am J Respir Crit Care Med 2000; 162:1277–84.

22. Misumi S, Lynch DA. Idiopathic pulmonary fibrosis/ usual interstitial pneumonia: imaging diagnosis, spectrum of abnormalities, and temporal progression. Proc Am Thorac Soc 2006;3(4):307–14.

23. Silva CI, Muller NL, Lynch DA, et al. Chronic hypersensitivity pneumonitis: differentiation from idiopathic pulmonary fibrosis and nonspecific interstitial pneumonia by using thin-section CT. Radiology 2008; 246(1):288–97.

24. McAdams HP, Erasmus J. Chest case of the day: Williams-Campbell syndrome. Am J Roentgenol 1995;165:190.

25. Kinsella D, Sissons G, Williams MP. The radiological imaging of bronchial atresia. Br J Radiol 1992;65: 681.

26. Jederlinic PJ, Sicilian LS, Baigelman W, et al. Congenital bronchial atresia: a report of 4 cases and review of literature. Medicine 1986;66:73–83.

27. Glassroth J. Pulmonary disease due to nontuberculous mycobacteria. Chest 2008;133:243–51.

28. Kuroishi S, Nakamura Y, Hayakawa H, et al. Mycobacterium avium complex disease: prognostic implication of high-resolution computed tomography findings. Eur Respir J 2008;32:147–52.

29. Kim JS, Tanaka N, Newell JD, et al. Nontuberculous mycobacterial infection—CT scan findings, genotype, and treatment responsiveness. Chest 2005; 128:3863–9.

30. Hansell DM. Bronchiectasis. Radiol Clin North Am 1998;36(1):107–28.

31. Loch C, Cuppens H, Rainisio M, et al. European epidemiologic registry of cystic fibrosis (ERCF): comparison of major disease manifestations between patients with different classes of mutations. Pediatr Pulmonol 2001;31:1–12.

32. Vikgren J, Johnsson AA, Flinck A, et al. High-resolution computed tomography with 16-row MDCT: a comparison regarding visibility and motion artifacts of dose-modulated thin slices and "step and shoot" images. Acta Radiol 2008;23:1–6.

33. Martinez S, Heyneman LE, McAdams HP, et al. Mucoid impactions: finger-in-glove sign and other CT and radiographic features. Radiographics 2008; 28:1369–82.

34. Brown DE, Pittman JE, Leigh MW, et al. Early lung disease in young children with primary ciliary dyskinesia. Pediatr Pulmonol 2008;43:514–6.

35. Bush A, Chodhari R, Collins N, et al. Primary ciliary dyskinesia: current state of the art. Arch Dis Child 2007;92:1136–40.

36. Morozov A, Applegate KE, Brown S, et al. High-attenuation mucus plugs on MDCT in a child with cystic fibrosis: potential cause and differential diagnosis. Pediatr Radiol 2007;37(6):592–5.

Imaging of Small Airway Disease (SAD)

Sudhakar N.J. Pipavath, MBBS, Eric J. Stern, MD*

KEYWORDS

• Small airways disease • Bronchiolitis
• High resolution computed tomography
• Follicular bronchiolitis • Panbronchiolitis

DEFINITION

Small airways are generally considered synonymous with those airways at the bronchiolar level and beyond, have a luminal diameter of less than 1 to 2 mm, and contain no cartilage in their walls. Although distinct, small airways disease (SAD) and bronchiolitis are often used interchangeably. The two types of bronchioles—membranous and respiratory—have distinct histology and function.[1] Membranous bronchioles are conducting airways, and respiratory bronchioles are noted to have alveoli and alveolar ducts.

ANATOMY OF THE SECONDARY PULMONARY LOBULE

Understanding the anatomy of the secondary pulmonary lobule is essential for understanding SAD successfully. The secondary pulmonary lobule (Fig. 1) is the smallest, irregular/polyhedral-shaped unit of the lung marginated by connective tissue.[2] The center of the lobule is supplied by a paired bronchiole and pulmonary arteriole branch, and the secondary pulmonary lobule is marginated by connective tissue—the interlobular septa, which contains pulmonary venules and lymphatic channels. The preterminal bronchiole supplies the secondary pulmonary lobule, also called the lobular bronchiole, which gives rise to approximately three terminal bronchioles. The terminal bronchioles end in respiratory bronchioles. Respiratory bronchioles have three order branches; the alveolar ducts, sacs, and alveoli succeed them. The respiratory bronchiole is both a conducting and gas exchange unit. The acinus is defined as a unit of the lung that is distal to the terminal bronchiole, and it typically measures 7 mm in diameter.

APPROACH TO EVALUATING AND DIAGNOSING SMALL AIRWAY DISEASE

Imaging signs of SAD can be direct or indirect. Two common direct signs are (1) centrilobular branching nodules that often appear as V- or Y-shaped and sometimes are referred to as "tree in bud" opacities (Fig. 2)[3] and (2) centrilobular or peribronchiolar ground glass opacities. A less common direct sign includes bronchiolectasis, a feature seen only relatively late and with chronic forms of SAD.

Air trapping is an indirect sign of bronchiolar disease. In the clinical setting of actively inflamed bronchioles, inflammation or mucous plugging leads to premature closure or complete obstruction, with air trapping as a consequence.[4] In the setting of mature obliterative (constrictive) bronchiolitis, the airway lumen is narrowed or obliterated, and the lobule is ventilated by collateral drift. It is not an issue of premature closure as in the setting of acute inflammation; the closure is typically fixed or permanent. To diagnose air trapping on CT, expiratory images are essential.[5] Although lobular and segmental air trapping is appreciable on inspiratory scans, lobar air trapping often requires expiratory scans performed with

Department of Radiology, University of Washington Medical Center, 1959 NE Pacific Street, # 357115, Seattle, WA, USA
* Corresponding author.
E-mail address: estern@u.washington.edu (E. J. Stern).

Radiol Clin N Am 47 (2009) 307–316
doi:10.1016/j.rcl.2009.01.002

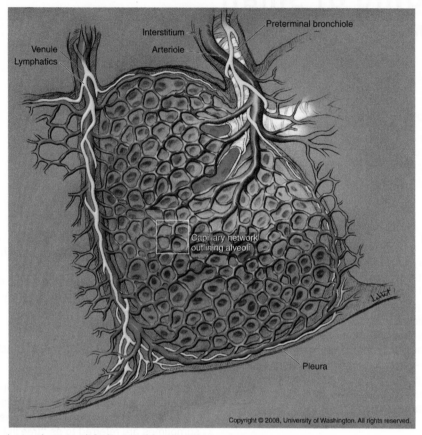

Fig. 1. Secondary pulmonary lobule. Line drawing with schematic depiction of secondary pulmonary lobule anatomy. (*Courtesy of* the University of Washington, Seattle, WA; with permission. Copyright © 2009 University of Washington.)

good patient effort. The most important confounder in diagnosing air trapping that results from SAD is the similar pulmonary mosaic attenuation pattern that results from pulmonary vascular disease. In other words, the mosaic attenuation pattern that results from SAD occurs in combination with the primary airway constriction and secondary hypoxic vasoconstriction. This is in contrast to the similar pattern of primary pulmonary vascular disease and associated secondary hypoxic bronchiolar constriction. Air trapping can be seen as a result of primary pulmonary vascular disease,[6] and possibly the original concept of being able to differentiate these two entities depends more on the associated abnormalities.

In the evaluation of patients who are suspected of having SAD, one should take into consideration the fact that some mild air trapping, mostly lobular, can be seen in otherwise normal healthy, nonsmoking individuals[7] and even in asymptomatic, otherwise healthy cigarette smokers. The extent of air trapping and associated clinical symptomatology helps in decision making.

INFLAMMATORY BRONCHIOLITIS
Infectious Bronchiolitis

Acute infections can cause inflammation of the small airways and a clinically severe form of lung dysfunction. Pathologically, epithelial necrosis, inflammation of the bronchiolar walls, and

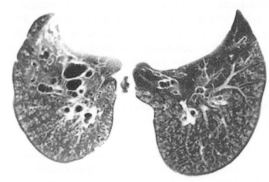

Fig. 2. Kartgener's syndrome. Axial HRCT images demonstrate fine centrilobular nodules and tree in bud pattern in the lower lobes with cystic and varicose bronchiectasis.

Table 1
Classification, causes, imaging features and differential diagnosis of SAD

Category	Type Based on Imaging or Pathologic Pattern	Prototype Cause and Other Causes	Imaging Features (HRCT)	Differential Diagnosis
Inflammatory				
—	Infectious	Viruses, mycoplasma, mycobacteria	Centrilobular nodules, tree in bud pattern, bronchial wall thickening, ground glass abnormality in a patchy distribution	Hypersensitivity pneumonitis, aspiration (in lower lung distribution)
	Respiratory bronchiolitis	Cigarette smoking	Centrilobular nodules and patchy ground glass opacities in an upper lung distribution	Hypersensitivity pneumonitis, pulmonary neovascularity in Eisenmenger's syndrome[27]
	Follicular bronchiolitis	Rheumatoid arthritis and Sjögren's syndrome	Lower lung dominant centrilobular and peribronchiolar nodules, bronchiolectasis and bronchiectasis	Asian panbronchiolitis, immunodeficiency syndromes, infectious bronchiolitis
	Asian panbronchiolitis	Idiopathic, relatively exclusive in patients of Asian origin	Lower lung bronchiectasis, bronchiolectasis, centrilobular nodules	Follicular bronchiolitis, immunodeficiency syndromes, and infectious bronchiolitis
Fibrotic bronchiolitis				
—	Constrictive or obliterative bronchiolitis	Postinfectious, Swyer-James Macleod syndrome, toxic fume inhalation	Patchy air trapping, bronchiectasis, and bronchiolectasis	Differential perfusion from pulmonary hypertension
	Obliterative bronchiolitis in postlung or hematopoietic stem cell transplant population	Postlung transplantation, chronic graft-versus-host disease	Lower lung dominant mosaic attenuation and air trapping with diminished vascularity	Postinfectious obliterative bronchiolitis

intraluminal exudation are seen in this setting. Acute viral infections are by far the most common infections to cause bronchitis and bronchiolitis. Although in children infectious bronchiolitis most frequently is the result of acute viral infections, in adults, viruses, mycoplasma, and bacteria are all equally responsible for acute infectious bronchiolitis. More chronic infections and nontuberculous and tuberculous mycobacterial infections can cause bronchiolitis. In immunosuppressed patients, causes for infectious bronchiolitis can include *Aspergillus* sp. cytomegalovirus, respiratory syncitial virus, and *Pseudomonas aeruginosa*.

Normal bronchioles at routine thin section imaging are not typically visible. When they become acutely or subacutely inflamed or filled with inflammatory exudate, they are much more likely to be visible[4] and demonstrate distinct sharply defined centrilobular nodules, centrilobular nodules with a "tree in bud" pattern, bronchiolar wall thickening, or indistinct, more ground glass–appearing centrilobular nodules, all with or without associated air trapping.[8] The secondary or indirect finding of air trapping occurs less frequently in acute infectious bronchiolitis. A feature that the authors have found useful in suggesting infectious etiology is the patchy distribution (**Fig. 3**). Noninfectious inflammatory bronchiolitis often has a more uniform and mostly bilateral or symmetric involvement (eg, in patients with Asian panbronchiolitis or follicular bronchiolitis). Associated areas of nonspecific ground glass opacities or even areas of focal or more dense consolidation may be seen in patients with infectious bronchiolitis. More extensive or chronic airway infections are much more likely to have associated bronchiectasis or bronchiolectasis (**Fig. 4**). If the pattern of bronchiolitis involves predominantly the right middle lobe and lingula, one should strongly consider mycobacterium avium intracellulare infection (**Fig. 5**), clinically the

so-called "Lady Windermere syndrome."[9] Colonization or superinfection of bronchiectatic airways with bacterial or nontuberculous mycobacteria cannot be differentiated from isolated infectious bronchiolitis alone (**Table 1**).

Smoking-related Small Airways Disease

Centrilobular emphysema, which falls under the broad category of chronic obstructive pulmonary disease, is not discussed in this article. This section focuses on respiratory bronchiolitis and respiratory bronchiolitis–associated interstitial lung disease (RB/RB-ILD). RB is mostly an asymptomatic condition seen in smokers. RB-ILD, however, is a form of interstitial pneumonia associated with RB. As the name suggests, cigarette smoking causes inflammation in and around the respiratory bronchioles. Hemosiderin-like pigment-laden macrophage accumulation within the respiratory bronchioles at pathology and ill-defined centrilobular nodules and, occasionally, centrilobular ground glass opacities at high resolution CT (HRCT) are common. RB-ILD tends to have more dominant interstitial inflammation and accumulation of hemosiderin-like pigment-laden macrophages in the alveolar spaces in addition to the respiratory bronchioles. At HRCT, RB-ILD manifests as dominant ground glass abnormality with centrilobular nodules (**Fig. 6**). Air trapping is not a common feature. RB and RB-ILD tend to have upper lung predominance.[10] Imaging differential diagnosis for RB includes infectious bronchiolitis and hypersensitivity pneumonitis. Hypersensitivity pneumonitis, desquamative interstitial pneumonia, and nonspecific interstitial pneumonitis are the imaging differential considerations for RB-ILD. Desquamative interstitial pneumonia has lower and peripheral lung dominant ground glass opacity. Well-defined cysts may be present within areas of ground glass opacity, a less sensitive but relatively more specific feature. Desquamative interstitial pneumonia

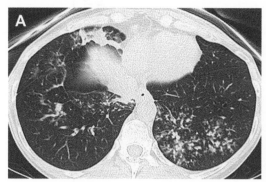
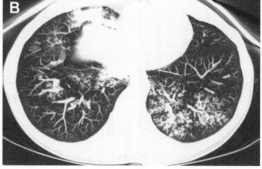

Fig. 3. Infectious bronchiolitis. A 37-year-old woman before matched unrelated peripheral blood stem cell transplant for AML, for a second transplant after relapsing after the first unrelated transplant. Axial HRCT (*A*) and MIP (*B*) images demonstrate patchy centrilobular nodules and tree in bud pattern, presumed to be bacterial infection.

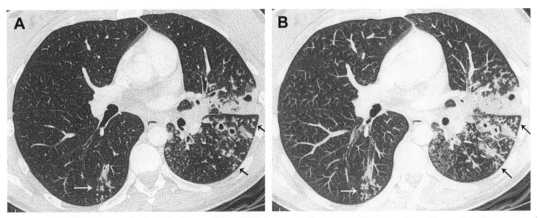

Fig. 4. Reactivation tuberculosis (Tb) with endobronchial spread of disease. (*A*) Thin collimation axial CT image and (*B*) MIP reformat demonstrate patchy centrilobular nodules and tree in bud appearance (*arrows*) in lower lobes and lingula. Bronchiectasis/bronchiolectasis is present in left lower lobe. (*Courtesy of* C. Beigelman-Aubry, MD, Paris, France.)

characteristically lacks centrilobular nodules that are otherwise common in RB-ILD.

Hypersensitivity pneumonitis has imaging features similar to RB and RB-ILD. Both demonstrate ill-defined centrilobular opacities and ground glass opacity (**Fig. 7**). Patients who develop hypersensitivity pneumonitis are usually nonsmokers, however, and smokers are thought to have some protective effect from developing hypersensitivity pneumonitis.[11]

Follicular Bronchiolitis

This is a form of bronchiolitis that results from hyperplasia of the lymphoid tissue around and along the small airways/bronchioles. It is classically associated with collagen vascular disease, specifically rheumatoid arthritis and Sjögren's syndrome. The lymphocytes are polyclonal on immunohistochemistry. On HRCT, centrilobular nodules, tree in bud, and peribronchial nodules

are dominant features,[12] whereas ground glass opacity is uncommon. A more common form of bronchiolitis seen in patients with rheumatoid arthritis is constrictive bronchiolitis (discussed in more detail later). There is also some association between treatment of rheumatoid arthritis with D-penicillamine therapy and occurrence of constrictive bronchiolitis.

FIBROTIC/CONSTRICTIVE BRONCHIOLITIS

Constrictive bronchiolitis, which is also known as obliterative bronchiolitis, is a category of disorders recognized by a pattern of peribronchiolar fibrosis resulting in complete cicatrization of bronchiolar lumen.[1] Although most commonly idiopathic, known causes include infections, toxic fume inhalation (oxides of nitrogen, chlorine), autoimmune disorders, including rheumatoid arthritis, graft-versus-host disease, lung transplantation, inflammatory bowel disease,[13] and drug reactions,

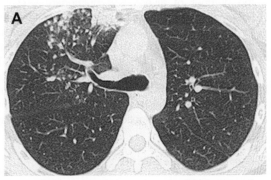
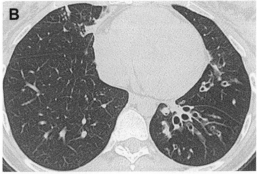

Fig. 5. Postinfectious bronchiectasis with bronchiolitis from super-added infection or colonization by mycobacterium avium intracellulare. Axial thin section CT demonstrates multiple centrilobular nodules in the right upper lobe and bronchiectasis in right middle lobe, lingual, and the left lower lobe.

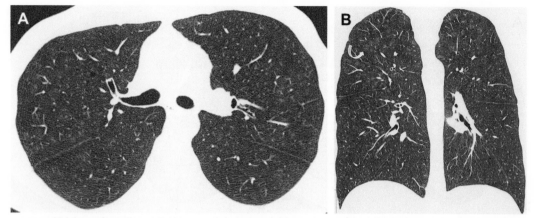

Fig. 6. Respiratory bronchiolitis from smoking. (*A*) Thin axial image and (*B*) coronal MIP reconstruction demonstrate multiple centrilobular ground glass opacities (*arrow, curved arrow*). (*Courtesy of* C. Beigelman-Aubry, MD, Paris, France.)

such as can be seen with D-penicillamine therapy. Direct CT signs of disease in and around airways are usually absent in this form of bronchiolitis. Bronchiectasis of larger airways can be associated. Air trapping as an indirect finding of airway narrowing/obliteration is the most common and identifying imaging feature of this broad category of bronchiolitis.

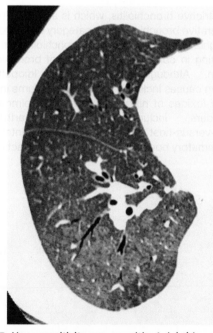

Fig. 7. Hypersensitivity pneumonitis. Axial thin section chest CT demonstrates multiple ill-defined centrilobular opacities (*arrow*). The image on the right from another patient demonstrates somewhat more discrete centrilobular nodules.

Postinfectious Constrictive Bronchiolitis

Pulmonary infections with agents such as adenovirus, measles, pertussis, mycoplasma, and tuberculosis can cause postinfectious bronchiolitis.[14] Postinfectious constrictive bronchiolitis also demonstrates mosaic attenuation/air trapping and rarely bronchiectasis or centrilobular nodules. As discussed earlier, infections and postinfectious constrictive bronchiolitis have a patchy distribution.[15]

Swyer-James or Macleod Syndrome

Swyer-James (or MacLeod) syndrome, a long-term complication of postinfectious constrictive bronchiolitis that occurs in childhood, is the development of unilateral hyperlucent lung with evidence of air trapping and decreased vascularity. Alveolar maturation occurs in children by the age of 8. Children who have infectious bronchiolitis before this age tend to either heal completely or heal with fibrosis, which affects alveolar maturation and results in a decrease in the number of alveoli and pulmonary vessels. Imaging of Swyer-James syndrome manifests as asymmetric patchy lobar or lobular air trapping that affects large areas. Originally this was thought to be unilateral and unilobar,[16] the advent of CT has made it increasingly clear that bilateral involvement is a rule rather than exception. Air trapping with diminished vascularity (Fig. 8), bronchiectasis, or hypoplastic lobe or lung is another typical feature.[17]

Noxious Fume Exposure

Exposure to various toxic fumes has been related to subsequent development of constrictive bronchiolitis. Initially some of these fumes may cause

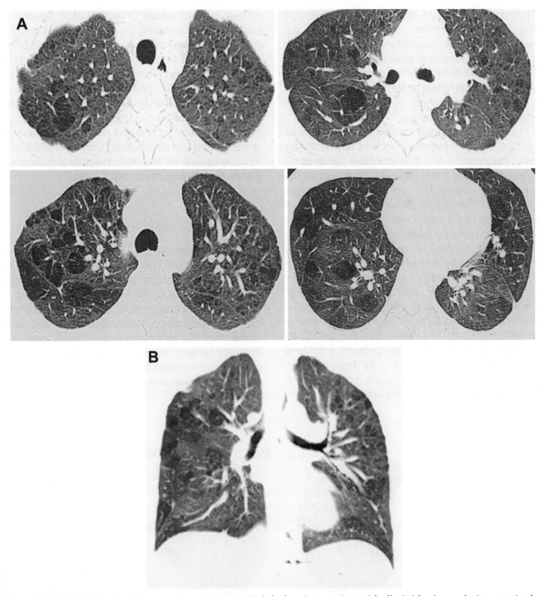

Fig. 8. (*A*) HRCT of the chest demonstrates asymmetric lobular air trapping with diminished vascularity seen in the lungs bilaterally from Swyer-James-Macleod syndrome. (*B*) Distribution of abnormality is better appreciated on the coronal reformatted image. (*Courtesy of* J.D. Godwin, MD, Seattle, WA.)

acute inflammatory disease. Imaging features are similar to other causes of constrictive bronchiolitis. Silo filler's lung from nitrogen dioxide exposure[18] and popcorn flavor manufacturing lung from di-acetyl exposure[19] are known to cause constrictive bronchiolitis. Post–nitrogen dioxide exposure bronchiolitis results from exuberant healing phase with formation of granulation tissue that accumulates at the site of the previous bronchiolar injury. Widespread obstruction and obliteration of small airways with or without associated peribronchiolar

fibrosis occurs as the healing progresses in 2 to 6 weeks.

Transplant-Related Bronchiolitis Obliterative Syndrome

Bronchiolitis obliterative syndrome can be defined as graft deterioration secondary to persistent airflow obstruction. Diagnosis does not necessarily require histologic confirmation; in contrast, the term "bronchiolitis obliterans" is used for a histologically proven diagnosis. This histologic diagnosis is restricted anatomically to the membranous and respiratory bronchioles and requires the presence of eosinophilic fibrous scarring of the wall of these small conducting airways with partial or complete obliteration of the lumen.[20] In advanced cases there is bronchial wall thickening and bronchiectasis.

At imaging, the presence of more than 32% air trapping has 87.5% sensitivity and specificity for the diagnosis of bronchiolitis obliterative syndrome, and in some patients this precedes the spirometric criteria for bronchiolitis obliterative syndrome.[21] Conversely, having less than 32% of air trapping has a high negative predictive value until the fifth postoperative year. In another, smaller study, an air-trapping score provided a sensitivity of 74% and a specificity of 67% for histopathologically proven obliterative bronchiolitis.[22] A more recent study, however, indicated that the value of the finding of air trapping in early stages of bronchiolitis obliterative syndrome is lower than was reported previously. The role of thin section CT as a screening test to evaluate patients with lung transplants was questioned.[23] Air trapping and, occasionally in advanced cases, bronchial wall thickening and bronchiectasis are seen (**Fig. 9**).[24]

Hyperpolarized helium (^{3}He) MRI is an upcoming tool that offers morphologic and functional assessment of lung ventilation and air trapping. It has been studied in post lung transplant patients. ^{3}He MRI has high spatial and temporal resolution compared with thin section CT, proton MRI, and radionuclide ventilation scan. The dynamic distribution of ventilation during continuous breathing after inhalation of a single breath of ^{3}He gas demonstrates homogeneous and fast distribution in normal individuals. In patients with air trapping, irregular and delayed patterns with redistribution are seen.[25]

ASIAN DIFFUSE PANBRONCHIOLITIS

Diffuse panbronchiolitis is an idiopathic chronic bronchiolitis seen most often in patients of Asian origin but is not limited to them. Imaging findings include centrilobular nodules, tree-in-bud, bronchiolectasis, bronchiectasis in a lower lobe with dominant distribution, which affects both the lower lobes (**Fig. 10**). Not surprisingly, mosaic attenuation may be seen on expiratory images.[26] Nonspecific patchy consolidation, mucoid impaction, and segmental atelectasis are some other imaging features.[15]

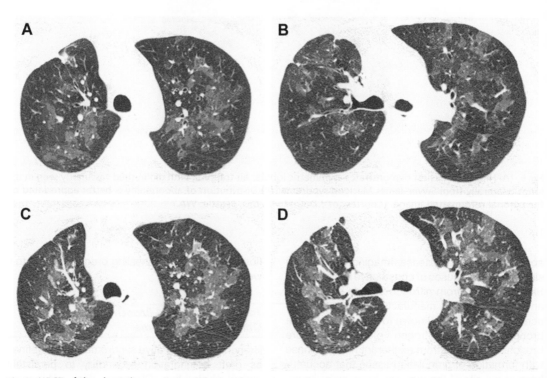

Fig. 9. HRCT of the chest demonstrates mosaic attenuation on inspiratory scans (*A, B*), with accentuation of the dark areas on expiratory scans (*C, D*) indicating severe air trapping in a patient with obliterative bronchiolitis from chronic graft-versus-host disease.

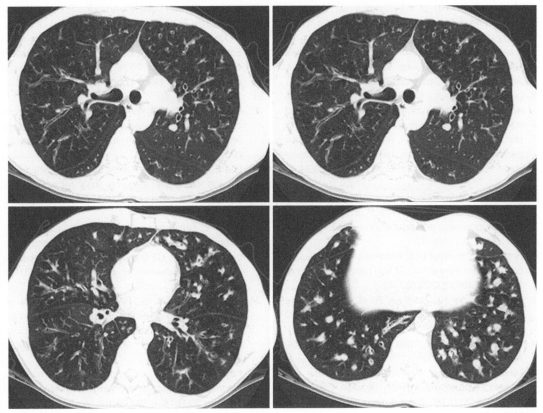

Fig. 10. Asian panbronchiolitis. HRCT images demonstrate bilateral relatively symmetric, lower lung dominant cylindrical bronchiectasis, bronchiolectasis, mucus plugging, and centrilobular nodules. (*Courtesy of* S. Young Kim, MD, Seoul, South Korea).

SUMMARY

The direct signs of SAD on CT include centrilobular nodules with or without "tree-in-bud" appearance and bronchiolectasis. Air trapping is an indirect sign of SAD and often needs expiratory imaging to diagnose it. Direct signs are often seen in patients with inflammatory bronchiolitis, and air trapping is a common feature in patients with fibrotic SAD. Infectious SAD tends to have a patchy appearance, whereas noninfectious SAD tends to be more uniformly distributed and relatively symmetric. Although most patients with SAD have overlapping features, a good clinical and radiologic interaction often helps narrow the imaging differential or arrive at a single diagnosis.

ACKNOWLEDGMENTS

The authors thank Professor J.D. Godwin for his guidance and support and Drs Catherine Beigelman-Aubry and Su Young Kim for invaluable images.

REFERENCES

1. Kuhn C III. Normal anatomy and histology. In: Thurlbeck WM, Churg AM, editors. Pathology of the lung. 2nd edition. New York: Thieme; 1995. p. 1–20.

2. Miller WS. The lung. Springfield (IL): Thomas; 1947. p. 39–42.

3. Collins J, Blankenbaker D, Stern EJ. CT patterns of bronchiolar disease: what is "tree-in-bud"? AJR Am J Roentgenol 1998;71:365–70.

4. Pipavath SJ, Lynch DA, Cool C, et al. Radiologic and pathologic features of bronchiolitis. AJR Am J Roentgenol 2005;185(2):354–63 [review].

5. Hansell DM. HRCT of obliterative bronchiolitis and other small airways diseases. Semin Roentgenol 2001;36(1):51–65.

6. Arakawa H, Stern EJ, Nakamoto T, et al. Chronic pulmonary thromboembolism: air trapping on computed tomography and correlation with pulmonary function tests. J Comput Assist Tomogr 2003; 27(5):735–42.

7. Mastora I, Remy-Jardin M, Sobaszek A, et al. Thin-section CT finding in 250 volunteers: assessment

of the relationship of CT findings with smoking history and pulmonary function test results. Radiology 2001;218(3):695–702.

8. Franquet T, Müller NL. Disorders of the small airways: high-resolution computed tomographic features. Semin Respir Crit Care Med 2003;24(4):437–44.

9. Levin DL. Radiology of pulmonary mycobacterium avium-intracellulare complex. Clin Chest Med 2002;23(3):603–12 [review].

10. Hansell DM, Nicholson AG. Smoking-related diffuse parenchymal lung disease: HRCT-pathologic correlation. Semin Respir Crit Care Med 2003;24(4):377–92.

11. Baldwin CI, Todd A, Bourke S, et al. Pigeon fanciers' lung: effects of smoking on serum and salivary antibody responses to pigeon antigens. Clin Exp Immunol 1998;113(2):166–72.

12. Howling SJ, Hansell DM, Wells AU, et al. Follicular bronchiolitis: thin-section CT and histologic findings. Radiology 1999;212(3):637–42.

13. Ward H, Fisher KL, Waghray R, et al. Constrictive bronchiolitis and ulcerative colitis. Can Respir J 1999;6(2):197–200.

14. Wohl ME, Chernick V. State of the art: bronchiolitis. Am Rev Respir Dis 1978;118:759–81.

15. Lynch DA. Imaging of small airways disease and chronic obstructive pulmonary disease. Clin Chest Med 2008;29(1):165–79, vii [review].

16. Müller NL. Unilateral hyperlucent lung: MacLeod versus Swyer-James. Clin Radiol 2004;59(11):1048.

17. Marti-Bonmati L, Ruiz Perales F, Catala F, et al. CT findings in Swyer-James syndrome. Radiology 1989;172(2):477–80.

18. Scott EG, Hunt WB Jr. Silo filler's disease. Chest 1973;63(5):701–6.

19. Martyny JW, Van Dyke MV, Arbuckle S, et al. Diacetyl exposures in the flavor manufacturing industry. J Occup Environ Hyg 2008;5(11):679–88.

20. Estenne M, Maurer JR, Boehler A, et al. Bronchiolitis obliterans syndrome 2001: an update of the diagnostic criteria. J Heart Lung Transplant 2002;21(3):297–310.

21. Bankier AA, Van Muylem AV, Knoop C, et al. Bronchiolitis obliterans syndrome in heart-lung transplant recipients: diagnosis with expiratory CT. Radiology 2001;218:533–9.

22. Lee ES, Gotway MB, Reddy GP, et al. Early bronchiolitis obliterans following lung transplantation: accuracy of expiratory thin-section CT for diagnosis. Radiology 2000;216:472–7.

23. Konen E, Gutierrez C, Chaparro C, et al. Bronchiolitis obliterans syndrome in lung transplant recipients: can thin-section CT findings predict disease before its clinical appearance? Radiology 2004;231(2):467–73.

24. Sargent MA, Cairns RA, Murdoch MJ, et al. Obstructive lung disease in children after allogeneic bone marrow transplantation: evaluation with high-resolution CT. AJR Am J Roentgenol 1995;164(3):693–6.

25. Kauczor HU. Hyperpolarized helium-3 gas magnetic resonance imaging of the lung. Top Magn Reson Imaging 2003;14(3):223–30 [review].

26. Nishimura K, Kitaichi M, Izumi T, et al. Diffuse panbronchiolitis: correlation of high-resolution CT and pathologic findings. Radiology 1992;184(3):779–85.

27. Sheehan R, Perloff JK, Fishbein MC, et al. Pulmonary neovascularity: a distinctive radiographic finding in Eisenmenger syndrome. Circulation 2005;112(18):2778–85.

Asthma: An Imaging Update

Alyn Q. Woods, MD[a,b,*], David A. Lynch, MB[a]

KEYWORDS

- Asthma • Radiology • CT • MRI • Imaging
- Synchrotron radiation • Hyperpolarized 3He

The incidence of asthma continues to increase worldwide, and in 2005 approximately 7.7% of the population of the United States (or 22.2 million individuals) carried the diagnosis.[1] Significant recent advances in imaging of asthma have yielded both a better understanding of the underlying pathophysiology as well as more effective assistance in guiding appropriate clinical therapy.

ASTHMA DEFINED

Asthma is characterized by all of the following:[2]

(1) airways obstruction that is usually reversible
(2) chronic airway inflammation, and
(3) nonspecific airways hyperreactivity.

The clinical diagnosis of asthma is most commonly made by documenting physiologic airway obstruction that improves following administration of bronchodilator. In more occult cases, asthma may be diagnosed by the presence of airway hyperreactivity to an inhaled substance, most commonly methacholine.

Beyond this basic definition, it is increasingly clear that asthma is heterogeneous with regard to its immunopathology, clinical phenotypes, natural history, and response to treatment. It was once considered to be an allergic disorder mediated by Th2-type lymphocytes, IgE, mast cells, eosinophils, macrophages, and cytokines. However, it is now evident that the pathophysiology of asthma also involves local factors such as local epithelial, mesenchymal, vascular, and neural structures.[3] These structural cells contribute to the development of a chronic asthma phenotype, with acute and subacute exacerbations being driven by environmental triggers, including allergens, microorganisms, and pollutants.

Rather than being a single disease entity, asthma seems to consist of related, overlapping syndromes.[4] Clinically important phenotypes of asthma include allergic asthma, aspirin-sensitive asthma, glucocorticoid-resistant asthma, and asthma with fixed airflow limitation.[4] Additionally, obese individuals may have a specific asthma phenotype, characterized by greater severity and poorer control with medications.[5] More recently, there is a suggestion that there is a phenotype of severe asthma characterized by air trapping visible on CT.[6]

Asthma may occur at any age, but most patients with asthma experience their first symptoms before age 5.[4] Most early-onset asthma has an allergic component.

Morphologically, asthma is characterized by airway remodeling, with infiltration of the airway wall by inflammatory cells, deposition of connective tissue, increase in smooth muscle mass, vascular changes, and hypertrophied mucous glands.[7–9] The airway remodeling of asthma is present by the age of 3.[10]

Asthma manifests clinically as periodic wheezing and shortness of breath. On physiologic evaluation, the forced expiratory lung volume in 1 second (FEV1) is reduced below 80% of normal, and the ratio of FEV1 to forced vital capacity (FVC) is less than 70%. The ratio of lung residual volume to the total lung capacity (RV/TLC) is increased. The clinical diagnosis of asthma is most commonly made by documenting physiologic airway obstruction

[a] Division of Radiology, National Jewish Health, 1400 Jackson Street, Denver, CO 80206, USA
[b] University of Colorado Denver, Radiology Academic Office, Mail Stop 8200, Building L15, Room 2414, 12631 East 17th Avenue, PO Box 6511, Aurora, CO 80045, USA
* Corresponding author. University of Colorado Denver, Radiology Academic Office, Mail Stop 8200, Building L15, Room 2414, 12631 East 17th Avenue, PO Box 6511, Aurora, CO 80045, USA.
E-mail address: alyn.woods@ucdenver.edu (A.Q. Woods).

Radiol Clin N Am 47 (2009) 317–329
doi:10.1016/j.rcl.2008.11.008

that reverses with bronchodilators. In more occult cases, asthma may be diagnosed by the methacholine challenge test: FEV1 is measured after inhalation of progressively increasing concentrations of methacholine to identify bronchial hyperreactivity.[11]

CONDITIONS ASSOCIATED WITH ASTHMA

Chronic rhinosinusitis has a well-established association with asthma[12] and the greater the degree of mucosal thickening the higher the likelihood of airway obstruction.[13] Extensive sinus mucosal thickening is more common in those with acute exacerbations of asthma than in those without exacerbations.[14] The degree of mucosal thickening appears to correlate with blood and sputum eosinophilia.[12] The relationship between sinus disease and asthma appears most marked in those with severe mucosal changes on CT scan, suggesting that the thickened sinus mucosa is a site of immunologic activity, which intensifies the atopic response in the airways.[15] Sinus CT is commonly performed to document the extent of sinus disease in asthma (Fig. 1). In these patients, appropriate pretreatment with antibiotics, mucolytic agents, nasal steroids, or nasal saline, is helpful to reduce or eliminate sinus changes caused by acute inflammation or infection.[15]

Similarly, there is an established relationship between gastroesophageal reflux disease (GERD) and asthma. Treatment of gastroesophageal reflux may reduce symptoms and physiologic impairment due to asthma.[16,17] Therefore, radiologic identification of signs of esophageal reflux such as esophageal wall thickening[18] may be helpful in asthmatic patients (Fig. 2).

IMAGING FEATURES
Chest Radiograph

The radiographic features of asthma are not particularly specific, but the most common abnormality is bronchial wall thickening, with hyperinflation the second most common (though less reliable) finding (Fig. 3).[19] Whereas some series identify hyperinflation radiographically in asthmatic patients up to 24% of the time,[20] it is uncommon to see marked hyperinflation in asthmatic patients who do not also have emphysema. Indeed, many patients with asthma have normal or reduced lung volumes even during acute exacerbations of their condition.

It is important to reduce the number of chest radiographs obtained in the clinical evaluation of known asthmatic patients, particularly children,[21] in whom radiation exposure has greater potential harm. Routine chest radiographs are not usually obtained in patients with asthma, except when there are atypical features, or there is concern for a complication. The indication for chest radiographs in asthma is open to debate. Tsai and colleagues[22] suggested guidelines for selective performance of chest radiographs in adult patients admitted with acute exacerbations of obstructive airway disease, proposing that chest radiographs should be performed only in patients who fulfill one or more of the following criteria: a clinical diagnosis of chronic obstructive pulmonary disease (as defined by the American Thoracic Society); a history of fever, or temperature more than 37.8°C; clinical or ECG evidence of heart disease; history of intravenous drug abuse; seizures; immunosuppression; evidence of other lung disease; or prior thoracic surgery. In a prospective study using these criteria, management was changed on the basis of the chest radiograph in 31% of the patients evaluated.[22] It is clear that use of guidelines and education can substantially reduce the use of chest radiographs in asthmatic patients.[23] Buckmaster and Boon[21] suggested that radiographs are unnecessary in those with known asthma and those who are improving with treatment, unless pneumothorax is suspected, or the patient is in the intensive care unit. In their study, the performance of unnecessary chest radiographs, identified by these criteria, was reduced substantially following implementation of an educational program.

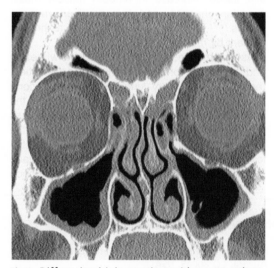

Fig.1. Diffuse sinusitis in a patient with severe asthma. Coronal CT shows mucosal thickening involving frontal, ethmoid and maxillary sinuses.

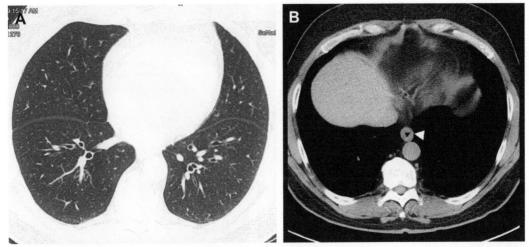

Fig. 2. Asthma with reflux esophagitis. (*A*) Axial CT shows moderate airway wall thickening. (*B*) Axial CT shows circumferential esophageal wall thickening (*arrowhead*).

CT

In patients with asthma, CT is indicated to identify suspected complications, particularly allergic bronchopulmonary aspergillosis, and mimics of asthma such as hypersensitivity pneumonitis. When it is performed, CT is helpful for evaluating the extent of airway thickening and expiratory air trapping (**Fig. 4**). Several studies using multidetector CT (MDCT) have clearly demonstrated the extent to which the airway walls of asthmatic patients are thicker than healthy individuals.[24] Furthermore, the degree of airway wall thickness directly correlates with the severity of airflow obstruction and clinical disease.[25,26]

A recent prospective study of CT in patients with asthma used automated quantitative 3-dimensional (3-D) CT analysis (**Fig. 5**) to show that airway wall thickness and area seen on MDCT correlated with airway epithelial thickness on endobronchial biopsy patients with severe asthma.[26] These authors also showed that patients with severe asthma have thicker airway walls on MDCT than mild asthmatic patients or healthy subjects, but overlap between these groups limits the diagnostic value of this measurement. As the authors acknowledge, a pivotal goal in those caring for individuals with severe asthma is to develop reliable and

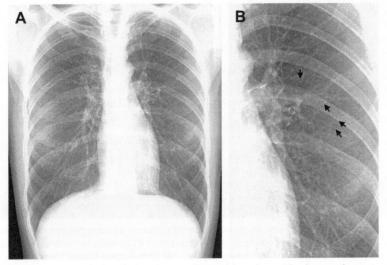

Fig. 3. (*A, B*) Chest radiograph with detail view in a patient with asthma. The lung volumes are increased, and there are numerous thick-walled airways around the hila (*arrows*).

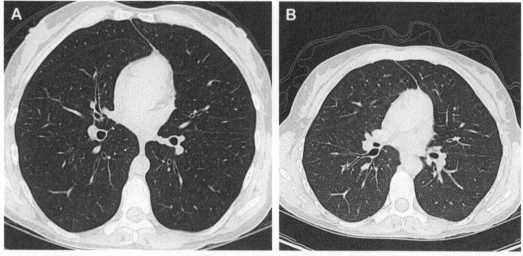

Fig. 4. CT findings in uncomplicated asthma (same patient as Fig. 3). (*A*) Inspiratory CT image shows diffuse airway wall thickening. (*B*) Expiratory CT shows diffuse air trapping.

reproducible yet noninvasive means to measure airway remodeling, which would allow providers both to identify those individuals more prone to develop severe disease as well as a means to effectively gauge the response to therapy. CT currently stands as the modality most likely to deliver this, and automated 3-D quantitative software will probably be the vehicle by which it is achieved.[27]

Air trapping can also be effectively quantified with CT, generally during expiration (**Fig. 6**).[28] A recent study by Busacker and colleagues[6] showed that quantitative CT cannot only determine air trapping in asthmatic subjects, but also identify a group of individuals with a high risk of severe disease. In this study, expiratory MDCT was performed in a subset of the subjects in the Severe Asthma Research Program. In this study, air trapping was defined as the percentage of lung less than −850 HU on expiratory CT, and those individuals with an air trapping percentage above the median value of 9.66% were defined as having an air-trapping phenotype. The threshold value of −850 was selected because the specific volume

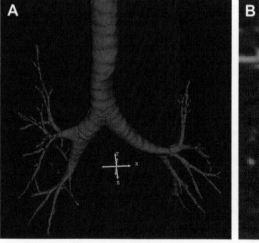
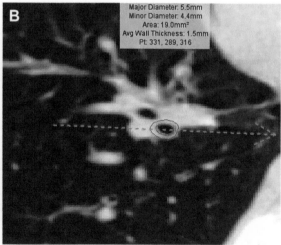

Major Diameter: 5.5mm
Minor Diameter: 4.4mm
Area: 19.0mm²
Avg Wall Thickness: 1.5mm
Pt: 331, 289, 316

Fig. 5. Quantitative analysis of airway wall thickening quantification in a young patient with severe asthma (FEV1/FVC ratio 0.59, residual volume 306% predicted). (*A*) Multidetector CT permits reconstruction of airway tree using proprietary software (VIDA Diagnostics Inc, Iowa City, IA). (*B*) Orthogonal image through the airway provides measurement of airway dimensions. The airways are moderately thick-walled. (*Courtesy of* Paul Szefler, Stanley Szefler, MD, and Ronina Covar, MD, National Jewish Health, Denver, CO.)

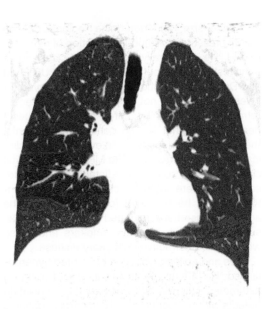

Fig. 6. Expiratory CT in asthma (same patient as Fig. 5). Coronal expiratory CT image shows moderate air trapping. Voxels with CT attenuation less than −856 Hounsfield Units are highlighted in color, with different colors for different lobes; 23% of the lung showed air trapping by this definition.

of the normal lung at total lung capacity is 6.0 mL/gm, corresponding to a CT attenuation of −856 HU. It seems reasonable therefore to assume that pixels with attenuation values less than this value represent persistently inflated lung on expiration. This threshold value has also been used to identify air trapping on single-slice CT in asthmatic children.[29] Using both univariate and multivariate statistical analysis, the clinical and demographic features of subjects with the air-trapping phenotype were compared with those without the phenotype. Individuals in the group with air trapping were significantly more likely to have a history of asthma-related hospitalizations, ICU visits, and/or mechanical ventilation. Duration of asthma, history of pneumonia, high levels of airway neutrophils, airflow obstruction (FEV(1)/FVC), and atopy were identified as independent risk factors associated with the air-trapping phenotype.[6]

Bronchial dilation, or bronchiectasis (defined as a bronchus with a larger diameter than the internal diameter of the adjacent pulmonary artery), has been well documented on CT in asthmatic patients (Fig. 7).[30–32] Lynch and colleagues[32] reported 77% of asthmatic patients had one or more dilated bronchi compared with 59% of healthy control subjects, whereas Park and colleagues[33] reported a prevalence of 31% in asthmatics and 7% in healthy controls. A study by Takemura and

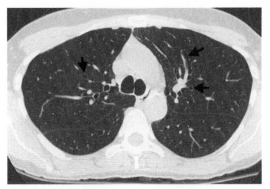

Fig. 7. Bronchial dilation in asthma. Inspiratory CT shows moderate dilation of central bronchi relative to adjacent vessels.

colleagues[30] confirmed that bronchial dilation is more prevalent in asthmatic patients than in healthy subjects, and like the study performed by Harmenci and colleagues,[31] they also suggest an association between an increased severity of asthma with a higher prevalence of bronchiectasis, as assessed by MDCT.

A difficult but important distinction for the radiologist and clinician is whether or not bronchiectasis observed in an asthmatic patient is associated with allergic bronchopulmonary aspirgillosis (ABPA). Although central bronchiectasis is important in the diagnosis of ABPA, the presence of dilated airways combined with an existing diagnosis of asthma should not automatically decree a diagnosis of ABPA. In fact, Neeld and colleagues,[34] and others,[35] have established that cylindric bronchiectasis can certainly be present without concomitant ABPA. Mitchell and colleagues[35] described the CT and radiographic findings in 19 patients with documented ABPA, 10 patients with probable ABPA, and 18 asthmatic controls without ABPA. All but one (89%) of the ABPA patients demonstrated central cystic or varicoid bronchiectasis in at least one lobe, and all 10 (100%) of the probable ABPA patients had evidence of bronchiectasis on HRCT, while 3 (17%) of the asthmatic controls had findings of cylindric bronchiectasis. In patients with asthma, CT imaging features that support the diagnosis of ABPA rather than asthma are varicose or cylindric bronchiectasis (Fig. 8),[35] mucoid impaction (see Fig. 8), and centrilobular nodules.[36] ABPA is further discussed elsewhere in this issue.

Synchrotron Radiation CT and Dual-Energy CT

While MDCT has good spatial resolution, and hyperpolarized ³He MR offers temporal resolution and quantitative measurements of functional lung parameters, some are investigating an innovative

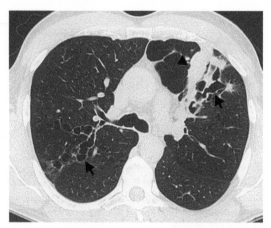

Fig. 8. Varicose bronchiectasis and mucoid impaction in allergic bronchopulmonary aspergillosis. CT shows marked dilation of multiple subsegmental airways (*arrows*) and mucoid impaction (*arrowhead*).

approach to effectively image both function and morphology simultaneously.[37] Synchrotron radiation CT using inhaled xenon as a contrast agent is an investigative technique pioneered by Bayat and colleagues[38] that appears preliminarily to fulfill these criteria. Their technique involves imaging with two monochromatic x-ray beams tuned to slightly different energies above and below the K-edge of xenon (Xe), with subsequent subtraction of the high-energy image from the low-energy image on a logarithmic scale, which subtracts the contributions of soft tissue and bone, yielding only the distribution of the contrast agent dispersed throughout the lungs.[38] Using this K-edge subtraction method (KES), Bayat and colleagues are able to quantitatively measure Xe contrast within the airways permitting the measurement of regional ventilation while also giving the high-resolution structural data. Future directions may include the simultaneous measurement of ventilation/perfusion maps using KES synchrotron CT imaging.[39] Current practical limitations include high radiation exposure, limited availability of synchrotron x-ray sources, and the requirement for the x-ray beam plane to remain stationary, requiring coordinated automated movement of the patient for image acquisition.[37] Similar techniques have been developed using dual-energy CT,[40] which is more widely available.

MR Imaging

Magnetic resonance (MR) imaging using hyperpolarized helium 3 (^{3}He) gas shows burgeoning promise in the evaluation of the lungs because of the ability to evaluate the spatial and temporal distribution of ventilation, quantitatively assess air space size, and determine regional oxygen partial pressure.[41] Although inhalation of hyperpolarized ^{3}He is generally safe, it is still classified as an investigational contrast agent by the US Food and Drug Administration and thus is approved for investigational, but not for clinical use. A recent retrospective study by Lutey and colleagues[41] demonstrated that in 100 consecutive patients, there were no serious adverse events and no clinically important effects of ^{3}He MR imaging on vital signs. Although some unpredictable transient desaturations were noted, which suggest that potential subjects be screened for comorbidities, the agent was used and tolerated not only in healthy subjects but also in heavy smokers and those with severe obstructive pulmonary disease.

Altes and colleagues[42] first presented hyperpolarized ^{3}He MR lung ventilation imaging findings in asthmatic patients, and showed that ventilation defects were present in 7 of 10 asthmatic patients but in none of 10 healthy subjects (**Fig. 9**). de Lange and colleagues[43] subsequently demonstrated that the amount of regional airflow obstruction depicted by hyperpolarized ^{3}He MR correlated with spirometric severity of asthma. The technique is very sensitive for identifying methacholine-induced air trapping.[44] In patients scanned on two occasions, ventilation defects identified with hyperpolarized ^{3}He were unchanged in location in about 40% of cases, and postmethacholine defects are unchanged in location in about 70% of cases, suggesting that the regional changes of asthma are relatively fixed within the lung.[44] Recent emphasis has focused on comparing the utility of hyperpolarized ^{3}He MR imaging against that of the established gold standard for airway evaluation, MDCT. Fain and colleagues[45] sought to compare regional ventilation defects in asthmatic patients on hyperpolarized ^{3}He MR with air trapping on MDCT and inflammatory makers on bronchoscopy. They found significant overlap of ventilatory defects on hyperpolarized ^{3}He MR with hyperlucency on MDCT, both of which correlated with elevated inflammatory markers (neutrophils) yielded by targeted bronchoalveolar lavage. Their findings again suggest that the areas of air trapping in the lungs of asthmatic individuals are relatively fixed. Tzeng and colleagues[46] used both hyperpolarized ^{3}He MR and MDCT to compare the airways of seven volunteers (five asthmatic, two healthy) before and after a methacholine challenge. Their technique yielded no meaningful correlation between the airway caliber changes measured on MR and MDCT. Airway measurement by hyperpolarized ^{3}He MR failed to match MDCT in 37% to 43% of the airway diameters from the first six generations

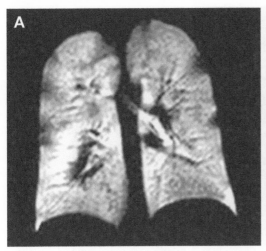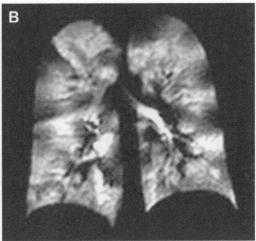

Fig. 9. Demonstration of ventilation defects by hyperpolarized ³He MR. (*A*) Coronal MR image in a mild-moderate asthmatic patient (FEV1 109% predicted) shows several small ventilation defects. (*B*) Follow-up image obtained after the patient was exposed to second-hand smoke, shows increase in number and size of ventilation defects. The FEV1 fell to 94% predicted, but remained within the normal range. (*Courtesy* of Dr Sean Fain, University of Wisconsin, Madison, WI.)

(at the two lung volumes tested, FRC and FRC + 1L). Although it may not yet rival the gold standard of MDCT because of poorer resolution and thus less anatomic detail, hyperpolarized ³He MR remains promising. In addition to providing greater patient safety because of the lack of ionizing radiation, the modality promises better functional physiologic data. Recent advances include those described by Wang and colleagues,[47] who have developed a novel hybrid MR pulse sequence that obtains coregistered maps of the apparent diffusion coefficient (ADC) of helium at both short and long time-scales (during a single breath hold). The ADC appears to be a sensitive method for detecting early alveolar destruction in emphysema,[48] and the study by Wang and colleagues[47] demonstrated significant elevations in ADC values in asthmatic patients compared with healthy controls suggesting that the alveolar spaces may also be expanded in asthma. Tsai and colleagues[49] have designed an open-access, low-field MR system for both horizontal and upright hyperpolarized ³He imaging of the human lungs, which has important physiologic implications given the limitations of some patients who are unable to remain horizontal for the required amount of time to be adequately imaged, as well as the inherent physiologic changes between the supine or prone lung with that of the upright lung. With continued advances in hyperpolarized ³He MR, widespread clinical use is possible, but may be limited by availability of ³He.

COMPLICATIONS OF ASTHMA

Radiologic imaging is important in identifying complications of asthma. Acute complications of asthma may include pneumothorax, pneumomediastinum (Fig. 10) (and rarely pneumopericardium, pneumoperitoneum, pneumoretroperitoneum, pneumorrhachis, and even subdural emphysema),[50–52] mucus impaction with or without atelectasis, and pneumonia.

Chronic complications of asthma include allergic bronchopulmonary aspergillosis (discussed elsewhere in this issue), eosinophilic pneumonia, and Churg-Strauss vasculitis. About 50% of patients with chronic eosinophilic pneumonia have a history of atopy, with or without asthma. The typical radiographic findings in chronic eosinophilic pneumonia are patchy airspace opacities, usually with upper lobe predominance. The peripheral distribution of the infiltrates may be evident on the chest radiograph as the "negative pulmonary edema pattern," but may be more obvious on CT scan.[53,54]

Churg-Strauss vasculitis (allergic granulomatosis and angiitis) is a granulomatous vasculitis that occurs in patients with asthma, and is commonly associated with eosinophilia. This vasculitis may also affect the skin, kidneys, and peripheral nerves. Pericardial or myocardial involvement may occur (Fig. 11).[55,56] CT shows lung parenchymal abnormalities in about 75% of cases.[57] Radiologically, it presents with patchy, often migratory consolidation or groundglass abnormality, often associated with airway wall

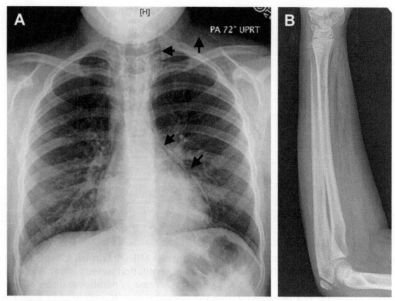

Fig. 10. Pneumomediastinum in a child with asthma. (A) Chest radiograph shows pneumomediastinum and air in the left neck (arrows). (B) Radiograph of left arm shows air in the soft tissues.

thickening and septal thickening (see **Fig. 11**).[58] Small nodules and tree-in-bud pattern may indicate bronchiolitis. The extrapulmonary involvement is often the main clue to the diagnosis. Churg-Strauss syndrome is usually more benign in its course than Wegener's granulomatosis.

MIMICS OF ASTHMA

The aphorism "all that wheezes is not asthma"[59] is most important for the radiologist. Any young person with breathlessness or wheezing may be assigned the label of asthma. Therefore, the challenge for the radiologist who reviews the images of a patient with "asthma" is to disprove this diagnosis. The most common condition to be misdiagnosed with asthma is vocal cord dysfunction, a functional condition in which inspiratory or expiratory stridor is produced by adduction of the vocal cords.[60] Patients with this disorder are often treated with large doses of steroids because of refractory asthma. The diagnosis of vocal cord

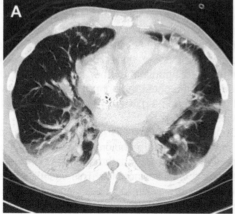
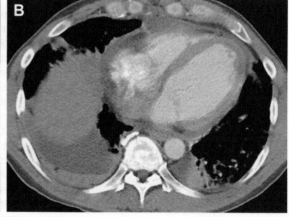

Fig. 11. Churg-Strauss syndrome in a 58- year-old man with a long history of asthma, and new fever and skin rash. (A) CT scan photographed at lung window settings shows bilateral basal predominant consolidation and ground-glass abnormality, with some peribronchovascular predominance. (B) CT photographed at lung windows at a lower level shows bilateral pleural effusions and a pericardial effusion. Left ventricle is mildly dilated because of cardiomyopathy.

dysfunction is made by laryngoscopy. There are no radiologic manifestations of vocal cord dysfunction, but one might suspect this condition when the chest radiograph or chest CT shows normal bronchial wall thickness in a patient who has severe symptoms.

Patients with tracheal or carinal obstruction commonly receive the label of asthma, in spite of the lack of fluctuation of their symptoms, and the frequent presence of inspiratory stridor (Fig. 12).[61] The obstructing airway lesion is often visible on the frontal or lateral chest radiograph, unless it is at the carina. Focal lesions causing tracheal obstruction include benign and malignant tracheal neoplasms, tracheal stenosis following intubation, and vascular rings.[62] Diffuse or long-segment tracheal narrowing may be a result of infiltrative disorders, such as sarcoidosis, Wegener's

granulomatosis, or amyloidosis, or may be caused by cartilaginous disorders, such as relapsing polychondritis or tracheobronchopathia osteochondroplastica. In patients with suspected tracheal obstruction, a flow-volume loop shows characteristic blunting of the inspiratory limb of the loop. Helical CT scan with multiplanar reformations or 3-D rendering can usefully define the surgical anatomy in these patients (see Fig. 12).[63]

Patients with constrictive bronchiolitis present with airway obstruction that is usually refractory to bronchodilators. Bronchiolitis in these patients may be a result of previous infection, collagen vascular disease, or may be idiopathic. It may be difficult or impossible to distinguish clinically between refractory, late-onset asthma and cryptogenic bronchiolitis obliterans. High-resolution CT scan assists with this distinction by identifying

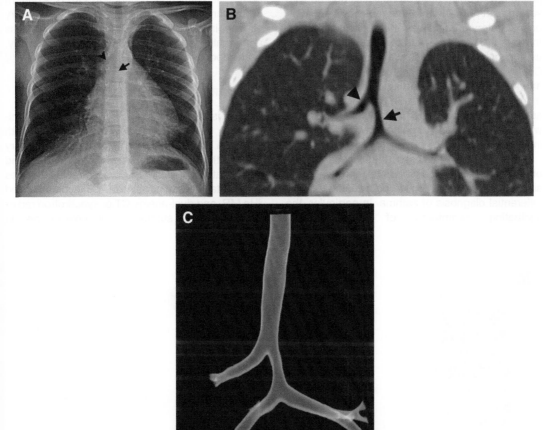

Fig. 12. Tracheal stenosis in a child with long-standing shortness of breath misdiagnosed as asthma. (A) Chest radiograph shows moderate tracheal narrowing just above the carina (arrow). A tracheal bronchus is also visible (arrowhead). (B, C) Coronal CT reconstruction and virtual bronchogram confirm these findings.

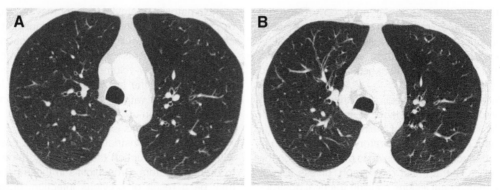

Fig. 13. Bronchiolitis obliterans. (*A*) Inspiratory CT shows decreased attenuation in the anterior left lung. (*B*) Expiratory CT shows air trapping in the same anterior distribution.

the sharply demarcated lobular areas of air trapping that are characteristic of cryptogenic bronchiolitis obliterans (**Fig. 13**). In a study of 14 patients with obliterative bronchiolitis and 30 with severe asthma, we found that mosaic attenuation on inspiratory images was the best discriminant, found in 50% of those with obliterative bronchiolitis and only one of those with severe asthma.[64] Copley and colleagues[65] found that vascular attenuation and decreased lung attenuation were more prevalent in obliterative bronchiolitis than in asthma. Patients with bronchiolitis obliterans who have diffuse air trapping, however, may be indistinguishable from those with asthma.

Infiltrative lung diseases that cause airway obstruction, such as sarcoidosis[66] and hypersensitivity pneumonitis,[67] must be included in the differential diagnosis of asthma. In particular, the fluctuating symptoms of hypersensitivity pneumonitis may closely mimic asthma. The peribronchiolar granulomas of hypersensitivity pneumonitis sometimes cause dominant airway obstruction rather than restriction. On CT, a pattern of lobular decrease in attenuation and expiratory air trapping, usually associated with groundglass abnormality and often with centrilobular nodularity, is an important clue to this diagnosis (**Fig. 14**).[68,69]

SUMMARY

Asthma is a common disease with increasing incidence, which manifests radiologically with common, but nonspecific findings. The primary task of the radiologist is to identify mimics and complications of asthma. However, rapid advances in quantitative imaging using MDCT, hyperpolarized ^{3}He MR, and dual-energy CT or synchrotron radiation CT with Xe subtraction all show promise in

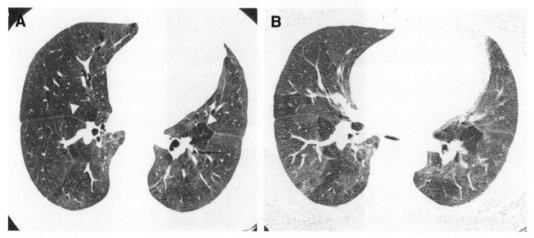

Fig. 14. Hypersensitivity pneumonitis in a patient presenting with "asthma." (*A*) Inspiratory CT shows patchy groundglass abnormality, with lobular decrease in lung attenuation (*white arrowheads*). (*B*) Expiratory CT shows multifocal air trapping.

improving the diagnosis and surveillance of the disease, which in turn should promote earlier recognition and guide more effective therapy.

REFERENCES

1. National Heart Lung and Blood Institute. 2007 NHLBI Morbidity and Mortality Chart Book. Available at: http://www.nhlbi.nih.gov/resources/docs/07-chtbk.pdf; 2008. Accessed January 15, 2009.

2. Guidelines for the diagnosis and management of asthma. Vol Publication No. 91–3042: National Asthma Education and Prevention Program.Department of Health and Human Services, Bethesda (MD);1991.

3. Holgate ST. Pathogenesis of asthma. Clin Exp Allergy 2008;38(6):872–97.

4. Kiley J, Smith R, Noel P, et al. Asthma phenotypes. Curr Opin Pulm Med 2007;13(1):19–23.

5. Lessard A, Turcotte H, Cormier Y, et al. Obesity and asthma: a specific phenotype? Chest 2008;134(2): 317–23.

6. Busacker A, Newell JD Jr, Keefe T, et al. A multivariate analysis of risk factors for the air-trapping asthmatic phenotype as measured by quantitative CT analysis. Chest 2009;135(1):48–56.

7. Carroll N, Elliot J, Morton A, et al. The structure of large and small airways in nonfatal and fatal asthma. Am Rev Respir Dis 1993;147(2):405–10.

8. Kay AB. Pathology of mild, severe, and fatal asthma. Am J Respir Crit Care Med 1996;154(2 Pt 2):S66–9.

9. James AL, Pare PD, Hogg JC, et al. The mechanics of airway narrowing in asthma. Am Rev Respir Dis 1989;139(1):242–6.

10. Bush A. How early do airway inflammation and remodeling occur? Allergol Int 2008;57(1):11–9.

11. Giannini D, Di Franco A, Bacci E, et al. The protective effect of salbutamol inhaled using different devices on methacholine bronchoconstriction. Chest 2000;117(5):1319–23.

12. Mehta V, Campeau NG, Kita H, et al. Blood and sputum eosinophil levels in asthma and their relationship to sinus computed tomographic findings. Mayo Clin Proc 2008;83(6):671–8.

13. Kim HY, So YK, Dhong H-J, et al. Prevalence of lower airway diseases in patients with chronic rhinosinusitis. Acta Oto-Laryngologica 2007;127(supp 558):110–4.

14. Peters EJ, Hatley TK, Crater SE, et al. Sinus computed tomography scan and markers of inflammation in vocal cord dysfunction and asthma. Ann Allergy Asthma Immunol 2003;90(3):316–22.

15. Phillips CD, Platts MT. Chronic sinusitis: relationship between CT findings and clinical history of asthma, allergy, eosinophilia, and infection. AJR Am J Roentgenol 1995;164(1):185–7.

16. Harding SM, Richter JE, Guzzo MR, et al. Asthma and gastroesophageal reflux: acid suppressive therapy improves asthma outcome. Am J Med 1996;100(4):395–405.

17. Peterson KA, Samuelson WM, Ryujin DT, et al. The role of gastroesophageal reflux in exercise-triggered asthma: a randomized controlled trial. Dig Dis Sci 2008. [Epub ahead of print].

18. Berkovich GY, Levine MS, Miller WT Jr, et al. CT findings in patients with esophagitis. AJR Am J Roentgenol 2000;175(5):1431–4.

19. Ismail Y, Loo CS, Zahary MK, et al. The value of routine chest radiographs in acute asthma admissions. Singapore Med J 1994;35(2):171–2.

20. Lynch DA. Imaging of asthma and allergic bronchopulmonary mycosis. Radiol Clin North Am 1998; 36(1):129–42.

21. Buckmaster A, Boon R. Reduce the rads: a quality assurance project on reducing unnecessary chest X-rays in children with asthma. J Paediatr Child Health 2005;41(3):107–11.

22. Tsai TW, Gallagher EJ, Lombardi G, et al. Guidelines for the selective ordering of admission chest radiography in adult obstructive airway disease. Ann Emerg Med 1993;22(12):1854–8.

23. Gentile NT, Ufberg J, Barnum M, et al. Guidelines reduce x-ray and blood gas utilization in acute asthma. Am J Emerg Med 2003;21(6):451–3.

24. Little SA, Sproule MW, Cowan MD, et al. High resolution computed tomographic assessment of airway wall thickness in chronic asthma: reproducibility and relationship with lung function and severity. Thorax 2002;57(3):247–53.

25. Niimi A, Matsumoto H, Amitani R, et al. Airway wall thickness in asthma assessed by computed tomography. Relation to clinical indices. Am J Respir Crit Care Med 2000;162(4 Pt 1):1518–23.

26. Aysola RS, Hoffman EA, Gierada D, et al. Airway remodeling measured by multidetector computed tomography is increased in severe asthma and correlates with pathology. Chest 2008;134(6): 1183–91.

27. Tschirren J, Hoffman EA, McLennan G, et al. Segmentation and quantitative analysis of intrathoracic airway trees from computed tomography images. Proc Am Thorac Soc 2005;2(6):484–7 503–4.

28. Newman KB, Lynch DA, Newman LS Jr, et al. Quantitative computed tomography detects air trapping due to asthma. Chest 1994;106(1): 105–9.

29. Jain N, Covar RA, Gleason MC, et al. Quantitative computed tomography detects peripheral airway disease in asthmatic children. Pediatr Pulmonol 2005;40(3):211–8.

30. Takemura M, Niimi A, Minakuchi M, et al. Bronchial dilatation in asthma: relation to clinical and sputum indices. Chest 2004;125(4):1352–8.

31. Harmanci E, Kebapci M, Metintas M, et al. High-resolution computed tomography findings are correlated with disease severity in asthma. Respiration 2002;69(5):420–6.

32. Lynch DA, Newell JD, Tschomper BA, et al. Uncomplicated asthma in adults: comparison of CT appearance of the lungs in asthmatic and healthy subjects. Radiology 1993;188(3):829–33.

33. Park CS, Muller NL, Worthy SA, et al. Airway obstruction in asthmatic and healthy individuals: inspiratory and expiratory thin-section CT findings. Radiology 1997;203(2):361–7.

34. Neeld DA, Goodman LR, Gurney JW, et al. Computerized tomography in the evaluation of allergic bronchopulmonary aspergillosis. Am Rev Respir Dis 1990;142(5):1200–5.

35. Mitchell TA, Hamilos DL, Lynch DA, et al. Distribution and severity of bronchiectasis in allergic bronchopulmonary aspergillosis (ABPA). J Asthma 2000;37(1):65–72.

36. Ward S, Heyneman L, Lee MJ, et al. Accuracy of CT in the diagnosis of allergic bronchopulmonary aspergillosis in asthmatic patients. AJR Am J Roentgenol 1999;173(4):937–42.

37. Bayat S, Porra L, Suhonen H, et al. Imaging of lung function using synchrotron radiation computed tomography: what's new? Eur J Radiol 2008;68(3):S78–83.

38. Bayat S, Le Duc G, Porra L, et al. Quantitative functional lung imaging with synchrotron radiation using inhaled xenon as contrast agent. Phys Med Biol 2001;46(12):3287–99.

39. Adam JF, Nemoz C, Bravin A, et al. High-resolution blood-brain barrier permeability and blood volume imaging using quantitative synchrotron radiation computed tomography: study on an F98 rat brain glioma. J Cereb Blood Flow Metab 2005;25(2):145–53.

40. Chae EJ, Seo JB, Goo HW, et al. Xenon ventilation CT with a dual-energy technique of dual-source CT: initial experience. Radiology 2008;248(2):615–24.

41. Lutey BA, Lefrak SS, Woods JC, et al. Hyperpolarized 3He MR imaging: physiologic monitoring observations and safety considerations in 100 consecutive subjects. Radiology 2008;248(2):655–61.

42. Altes TA, Powers PL, Knight-Scott J, et al. Hyperpolarized 3He MR lung ventilation imaging in asthmatics: preliminary findings. J Magn Reson Imaging 2001;13(3):378–84.

43. de Lange EE, Altes TA, Patrie JT, et al. Evaluation of asthma with hyperpolarized helium-3 MRI: correlation with clinical severity and spirometry. Chest 2006;130(4):1055–62.

44. de Lange EE, Altes TA, Patrie JT, et al. The variability of regional airflow obstruction within the lungs of patients with asthma: assessment with hyperpolarized helium-3 magnetic resonance imaging. J Allergy Clin Immunol 2007;119(5):1072–8.

45. Fain SB, Gonzalez-Fernandez G, Peterson ET, et al. Evaluation of structure-function relationships in asthma using multidetector CT and hyperpolarized He-3 MRI. Acad Radiol 2008;15(6):753–62.

46. Tzeng YS, Hoffman E, Cook-Granroth J, et al. Investigation of hyperpolarized 3He magnetic resonance imaging utility in examining human airway diameter behavior in asthma through comparison with high-resolution computed tomography. Acad Radiol 2008;15(6):799–808.

47. Wang C, Altes TA, Mugler JP 3rd, et al. Assessment of the lung microstructure in patients with asthma using hyperpolarized 3He diffusion MRI at two time scales: comparison with healthy subjects and patients with COPD. J Magn Reson Imaging 2008;28(1):80–8.

48. Fain SB, Panth SR, Evans MD, et al. Early emphysematous changes in asymptomatic smokers: detection with 3He MR imaging. Radiology 2006;239(3):875–83.

49. Tsai LL, Mair RW, Rosen MS, et al. An open-access, very-low-field MRI system for posture-dependent 3He human lung imaging. J Magn Reson 2008;193(2):274–85.

50. van der Klooster JM, Grootendorst AF, Ophof PJ, et al. Pneumomediastinum: an unusual complication of bronchial asthma in a young man. Neth J Med 1998;52(4):150–4.

51. Caramella D, Bulleri A, Battolla L, et al. Spontaneous epidural emphysema and pneumomediastinum during an asthmatic attack in a child. Pediatr Radiol 1997;27(12):929–31.

52. Sekiya K, Hojyo T, Yamada H, et al. Pneumoperitoneum recurring concomitantly with asthmatic exacerbation. Intern Med 2008;47(1):47–9.

53. Mayo JR, Muller NL, Road J, et al. Chronic eosinophilic pneumonia: CT findings in six cases. AJR Am J Roentgenol 1989;153:727–30.

54. Jeong YJ, Kim KI, Seo IJ, et al. Eosinophilic lung diseases: a clinical, radiologic, and pathologic overview. Radiographics 2007;27(3):617–37.

55. Matsuo S, Sato Y, Matsumoto T, et al. Churg-Strauss syndrome presenting with massive pericardial effusion. Heart Vessels 2007;22(2):128–30.

56. Vallejo E, Mendoza-Gonzalez C, Aranda A, et al. Churg-Strauss syndrome and myocardial perfusion SPECT imaging. J Nucl Cardiol 2004;11(3):358–60.

57. Kim YK, Lee KS, Chung MP, et al. Pulmonary involvement in Churg-Strauss syndrome: an analysis of CT, clinical, and pathologic findings. Eur Radiol 2007;17(12):3157–65.

58. Silva CI, Muller NL, Fujimoto K, et al. Churg-Strauss syndrome: high resolution CT and pathologic findings. J Thorac Imaging 2005;20(2):74–80.

59. Goldman J. All that wheezes is not asthma. Practitioner 1997;241(1570):35–8.

60. Hicks M, Brugman SM, Katial R, et al. Vocal cord dysfunction/paradoxical vocal fold motion. Prim Care 2008;35(1):81–103, vii.

61. Mehra PK, Woessner KM. Dyspnea, wheezing, and airways obstruction: is it asthma? Allergy Asthma Proc 2005;26(4):319–22.
62. McSharry DG, McElwaine P, Segadal L, et al. All that wheezes is not asthma. Lancet 2007;370(9589):800.
63. Boiselle PM, Reynolds KF, Ernst A, et al. Multiplanar and three-dimensional imaging of the central airways with multidetector CT. AJR Am J Roentgenol 2002;179(2):301–8.
64. Jensen SP, Lynch DA, Brown KK, et al. High-resolution CT features of severe asthma and bronchiolitis obliterans. Clin Radiol 2002;57(12): 1078–85.
65. Copley SJ, Wells AU, Muller NL, et al. Thin-section CT in obstructive pulmonary disease: discriminatory value. Radiology 2002;223(3):812–9.
66. Bartz RR, Stern EJ. Airways obstruction in patients with sarcoidosis: expiratory CT scan findings. J Thorac Imaging 2000;15(4):285–9.
67. Hansell DM, Wells AU, Padley SP, et al. Hypersensitivity pneumonitis: correlation of individual CT patterns with functional abnormalities. Radiology 1996;199(1):123–8.
68. Silva CI, Churg A, Muller NL, et al. Hypersensitivity pneumonitis: spectrum of high-resolution CT and pathologic findings. AJR Am J Roentgenol 2007; 188(2):334–44.
69. Silva CI, Muller NL, Lynch DA, et al. Chronic hypersensitivity pneumonitis: differentiation from idiopathic pulmonary fibrosis and nonspecific interstitial pneumonia by using thin-section CT. Radiology 2008;246(1):288–97.

Imaging of Airways: Chronic Obstructive Pulmonary Disease

Julia Ley-Zaporozhan, MD[a],*, Hans-Ulrich Kauczor, MD, PhD[b]

KEYWORDS

- COPD • Airways • CT • MRI • Visualization • Quantification

Chronic obstructive pulmonary disease (COPD) is one of the leading causes of morbidity and mortality worldwide. At present, it is the fourth most common cause of death among adults.[1] COPD is characterized by airflow limitation that is not fully reversible. The airflow limitation is usually progressive and associated with an abnormal inflammatory response of the lung to noxious particles or gases. It is caused by a mixture of airway obstruction (obstructive bronchiolitis) and parenchymal destruction (emphysema), the relative contributions of which are variable.[1] Chronic bronchitis, or the presence of cough and sputum production for at least 3 months in each of 2 consecutive years, remains a clinically and epidemiologically useful term. Pulmonary emphysema is a pathologic term and is defined by the American Thoracic Society as an abnormal permanent enlargement of the air spaces distal to the terminal bronchiole, accompanied by the destruction of their walls.[2] In a simplified way, obstructive airflow limitation leads to air trapping with subsequent hyperinflation and later destruction of the lung parenchyma.

For diagnosis and severity assessment pulmonary function tests (PFT) are the accepted and standardized workhorse providing quantitative measures for forced expiration volume in one second (FEV$_1$), FEV$_1$/FVC (forced vital capacity), diffusing capacity for carbon monoxide (DLco) and others. However, PFT only provide a global measure without any regional information not to mention any detail about lung structure. Although

extremely useful, PFTs are known to be relatively insensitive to both early stages and small changes of manifest disease.

The manifestations of obstructive lung disease are not limited to the tracheobronchial tree, but also affect the parenchyma by hyperinflation and destruction; as well as the vasculature by hypoxic vasoconstriction. Several pathologic studies have shown that a major site of airway obstruction in patients with COPD is in airways smaller than 2 mm of internal diameter.[3] The 2-mm airways are located between the fourth and the 14th generation of the tracheobronchial tree. Airflow limitation is closely associated with the severity of luminal occlusion by inflammatory exudates and thickening of the airway walls due to remodeling.[4]

COPD obviously comprises several subtypes which primarily can be related to the major site of involvement and then further differentiated. The subtypes include the airways, mainly obstructive bronchiolitis, and the parenchyma (ie, emphysema). PFTs, as a global measure, are unable to categorize these subtypes. With the increasing number of therapeutic options in COPD, particularly in its advanced stages, there is a high demand for a noninvasive imaging test to identify different phenotypes of the disease according to structural and functional changes and provide the regional information of such changes to target therapies accordingly. For phenotyping, a precise characterization of the different components of the disease, such as inflammation, hyperinflation,

[a] Department of Diagnostic and Interventional Radiology, University Hospital Heidelberg, Im Neuenheimer Feld 430, 69120 Heidelberg, Germany
[b] Department of Diagnostic and Interventional Radiology, University Hospital Heidelberg, Im Neuenheimer Feld 150, 69120 Heidelberg, Germany
* Corresponding author.
E-mail address: julia.leyzaporozhan@gmail.com (J. Ley-Zaporozhan).

Radiol Clin N Am 47 (2009) 331–342
doi:10.1016/j.rcl.2008.11.012
0033-8389/08/$ – see front matter © 2009 Elsevier Inc. All rights reserved.

and so forth, is highly desirable to select the appropriate therapy.

In contrast to PFT, radiological imaging techniques might allow for differentiation of the different components of obstructive lung disease (ie, airways, parenchyma, and vasculature) on a regional basis. Computed tomography (CT) is a long standing player in this field with emphasis on structural imaging of lung parenchyma and airways. Magnetic resonance imaging (MR imaging) of the lung has the potential to provide regional information about the lung without the use of ionizing radiation, but is hampered by several challenges: the low amount of tissue relates to a small number of protons leading to low signal, countless air-tissue interfaces cause substantial susceptibility artifacts as well as respiratory and cardiac motion.[5,6] The strength of MR imaging is the assessment of function like perfusion, ventilation, and respiratory dynamics.

This overview focuses on the imaging of the airway component of COPD. Enlarged or thickened airways can be directly visualized while pathologies of the small airways are frequently assessed by indirect signs like expiratory air trapping.

COMPUTED TOMOGRAPHY
Technical Aspects

At the present time, a state of the art multidetector computed tomography of the thorax yields a volumetric dataset of images with an isotropic submillimeter resolution (0.5 to 0.75 mm slice thickness). It covers the complete thoracic cavity in a single breath hold. CT can characterize anatomic details of the lung as small as 200 μm to 300 μm, which corresponds to approximately the seventh to ninth bronchial generation.[7] Since normal centrilobular bronchioles are not visible at thin-section CT, the recognition of air-filled airways in the lung periphery usually means that the airways are both dilated and thick-walled. The combination of high spatial resolution and volumetric coverage of the lung is recommended as it results in three-dimensional high resolution CT (3D HRCT). For multiplanar reformats, and other post processing tools, overlapping reconstruction is advantageous. The reconstructed slice thickness should match the collimation and the reconstruction increment and should be 80% of the slice thickness or less. Using a 512 or 768 matrix and a small reconstruction field of view targeted onto the tracheobronchial tree, the spatial resolution can be further optimized. Thin slices inherently carry a high level of image noise. Together with image reconstruction using a high-spatial resolution

kernel, noisy images might result. The trade-off between high-resolution images, which is what we are used to from traditional HRCT, and noise currently poses a major challenge. The detailed visual assessment of small structures, such as peripheral airways in the lung parenchyma, normally requires a high-resolution kernel. At the same time, the performance of postprocessing segmentation and quantitation using dedicated software tools is often hampered by noisy high-resolution images. The use of images reconstructed with a regular soft tissue kernel might be more appropriate.[8,9] As the airways in the lung parenchyma are high contrast structures, intermediate dose settings are appropriate. In general, a tube voltage of 120 kV together with a tube current between 50 mAs to 150 mAs is recommended.

Visualization of Large Airways

The isotropic datasets allow for different postprocessing techniques to be used for evaluation and presentation purposes.[10,11] Two different techniques are generally used and described later in this article: (1) two-dimensional multiplanar reformats (MPR), which allows assessment of the central airways along their anatomic course and reduction of the number of images to be analyzed; (2) complex three-dimensional segmentations and volume rendering which illustrate the important findings in a very intuitive way (eg, a frontal view of the patient or a simulation of an intraoperative situs) although they are more time consuming. Owing to this capability for continuous volumetric acquisitions during a single breath hold, multislice CT has developed as the gold standard for visualization of intra- and extraluminal pathology of the trachea and the bronchi. A presentation of overlapping thin slices in a cine mode allows identifying the bronchial divisions from the segmental origin down to the small airways. This viewing technique helps to identify intraluminal lesions, characterize the distribution pattern of any airway disease, and might also serve as a road map for the bronchoscopist. The perception of the anatomy of the tracheobronchial tree is further enhanced by MPR and maximal, and especially, minimal intensity projections. Interactive viewing of MPR on a workstation is the best way to find the appropriate plane in which key features of the disease are displayed. These views allow to confidently identify the main pattern of the disease, any associated findings, and the distribution of lesions relative to the airways. Tracheobronchial stenoses, especially in the vertically oriented bronchi, are often underestimated if evaluated on axial slices only.[12] MPR allow obviating this underestimation as the craniocaudal extension can be exactly determined. Beyond the assessment of the extent of stenosis, MPR are of value in treatment planning and follow-up as well as quantification of pathologic changes in obstructive lung disease like bronchial wall thickening.[13]

The maximum intensity projection (MIP) technique projects the highest attenuation value of the voxels on each view throughout the volume onto a two-dimensional image.[14] This method does not change the high resolution of the thin slices. Since the bronchiolar walls measure less than 0.1 mm in thickness, the small airways are normally not visible on volumetric high-resolution CT. However, when inflammatory changes are present in the bronchiolar wall and lumen, the bronchioles may become visible on CT scans, as small centrilobular nodular or linear opacities. The application of the MIP technique with the generation of 4- to 7-mm thick slabs may increase the detection and improve the visualization of these small centrilobular opacities.[12,15,16]

The minimum intensity projections (minIP) are a simple form of volume rendering to visualize the tracheobronchial air column into a single viewing plane. It is usually applied to a selected subvolume of the lung which contains the airways under evaluation. The pixels encode the minimum voxel density encountered by each ray. Subsequently, an airway is visualized because the air contained within the tracheobronchial tree has a lower attenuation than the surrounding pulmonary parenchyma. This technique displays only 10% of the data set and is the optimal tool for the detection, localization, and quantification of ground-glass and linear attenuation patterns.[14] In clinical routine, minIP are rarely used in the evaluation of the airways because numerous drawbacks have limited its indications in the assessment of airway disease. The technique is especially susceptible to variable densities within the volume of interest and partial volume effects.[12]

Three-dimensional surface rendering techniques and volume rendering techniques are very helpful to enhance the visualization of the anatomy of the airway tree. CT bronchography consists of a volume-rendering technique applied at the level of central airways after reconstruction of 3D images of the air column contained in the airways. Virtual bronchoscopy provides an internal analysis of the tracheobronchial walls and lumen owing to a perspective rendering algorithm that simulates an endoscopic view of the internal surface of the airways. In comparison to bronchoscopy, CT allows for visualization beyond stenoses, which supports planning of endobronchial procedures.[17]

Thus, virtual bronchoscopy can be extremely helpful in a clinical setting, especially in planning transbronchial biopsies.

Assessment of Small Airways Disease

To assess the presence of expiratory obstruction, multislice CT acquisitions in inspiration and expiration are recommended; especially for the acquisition of the expiratory scan, a low mAs protocol, 40- to 80- mAs, will be sufficient.[18] Regional air trapping reflects the retention of excess gas at any stage of respiration as an indirect sign of peripheral airway obstruction, predominantly seen on expiratory images. At expiration, the cross section of the lung will decrease, together with an increase of lung attenuation. Usually, gravity dependent areas will show a greater increase in lung density during expiration than nondependent lung regions. At the same time, the cross-sectional area of the airways will also decrease. Air trapping is defined as the lack of an increase of lung attenuation and the decrease of the cross-sectional area of lung. Air trapping may be depicted in individual lobes in the dependent regions of the lung. In general, any air trapping involving less than 25% of the cross-sectional area of one lung at a single scan level can still be regarded as a physiologic finding. Thus, physiologic air trapping will be detected at an expiratory CT in up to 50% of asymptomatic subjects. The frequency of air trapping will increase with age and is also associated with smoking.[19] Some publications suggest that the extent of air trapping is related to smoking history independent from the current smoking habits. Air trapping has to be considered pathologic when it affects a volume of lung equal or greater than a pulmonary segment, and not limited to the superior segment of the lower lobe.[20] Abnormal air trapping is a hallmark of small airway disease but it may also be seen in a variety of lung diseases, including emphysema, bronchiectasis, bronchiolitis obliterans, and asthma.[21]

Qualitative Evaluation

Trachea

Tracheobronchomalacia (TBM) generally results from weakness of the tracheal or mainstem bronchial walls caused by either softening of the supporting cartilaginous rings, redundancy of the connective tissue of the posterior membrane due to a reduction in the size and number of elastic fibers, or both. In association with COPD, TBM is usually diffusely distributed affecting the whole trachea. During exhalation, increasing pleural pressure causes the weakened central airways to narrow (collapse), which may exacerbate obstructive symptoms.[22] Symptoms can mimic worsening asthma or COPD, and it is not generally known which patients with COPD have TBM contributing to their symptoms. Acquired TBM has been reported in up to 44% of patients undergoing bronchoscopy in the setting of chronic bronchitis.[23] By consensus, excessive narrowing (collapse) is defined as a decrease of at least 50% in tracheal diameter during forced exhalation. For assessment of TBM cine acquisitions during continuous respiration or forced expiration (Fig. 1) by CT are recommended and easy to be performed.[24,25]

Large airways
Throughout the lung, the bronchi and pulmonary arteries run and branch together. The ratio of the size of the bronchus to its adjacent pulmonary artery is widely used as a criterion for detection of abnormal bronchial dilatation. In a healthy lung it should be the same at any level with the mean ratio being 0.98 [0.14] (with a wide range of 0.53–1.39).[26] The ratio of the internal luminal diameter of the bronchus to the diameter of its accompanying pulmonary artery has been estimated for the healthy subjects to be 0.62 [0.13].[27] CT signs of bronchiectasis are nontapering, or flaring, of bronchi, dilatation of the bronchi with or without bronchial wall thickening (signet ring sign), mucus-filled dilated bronchi (flame and blob sign), plugged and thickened centrilobular bronchioles (tree-in-bud sign), crowding of bronchi with associated volume loss, and areas of decreased attenuation reflecting small airways obliteration (Figs. 2 and 3).[28] The bronchiectasis are categorized in cylindric (mild bronchial dilatation, regular outline of the airway), varicose (greater bronchial dilatation, accompanied by local constrictions resulting in an irregular outline of the airway), and cystic or saccular type (ballooned appearance of the airways, reduced number of bronchial divisions).

Abnormalities of bronchial cartilage are also frequently present in COPD, associating atrophy and scarring. This deficiency of bronchial cartilage induces alternated narrowing and dilatation of the airways in advanced disease. This explains both, loss of normal proximal to distal tapering of the airway lumen and the presence of bronchiectasis in COPD patients. Like the trachea, collapse of segmental or subsegmental bronchi occurs at dynamic maximum forced expiratory maneuver due to cartilage deficiency.

Small airways
Small airways disease on CT can be categorized into visible and indirect patterns of the disease. The tree-in-bud sign reflects the presence of dilated centrilobular bronchioles with lumina that are impacted with mucus, fluid, or pus; it is often associated with peribronchiolar inflammation.[29] Cicatricial scarring of many bronchioles results in the indirect sign of patchy density differences of the lung parenchyma, reflecting areas of underventilation and air trapping and subsequent hypoperfusion (mosaic perfusion).

As a powerful adjunct to inspiratory scans, expiratory acquisitions reveal changes in lung attenuation related to air trapping and pulmonary blood volume, and illustrate regional volumetric

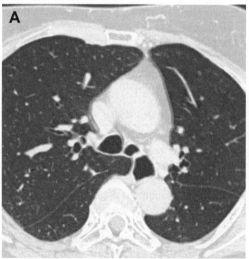
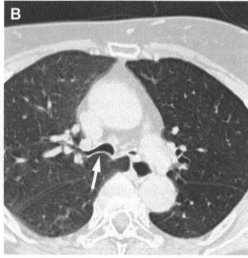

Fig. 1. CT images of a COPD patient at inspiration (A) and expiration (B) showing increased collapsibility of the right main bronchi (arrow) after exhalation due to bronchomalacia.

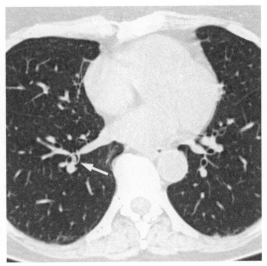

Fig. 2. Mucoid impaction in the lumen of the right lower lobe bronchus (segment 10, *arrow*).

changes providing deeper insights into local hyperinflation and expiratory obstruction (Fig. 4).[30] Since the severity of emphysema, as evaluated by CT, does not necessarily show a good correlation with FEV_1,[30,31] small airway disease appears to contribute more significantly to the airflow limitation in COPD. Regional air trapping reflects the retention of excess gas at any stage of respiration as an indirect sign of peripheral airway obstruction. It is best detected on expiratory CT as areas with abnormally low attenuation.[32] Air trapping is highly unspecific as it occurs under physiologic conditions as well as in a variety of lung diseases, including emphysema, bronchiectasis, bronchiolitis obliterans, and asthma.[21]

Quantitative Evaluation

Manual assessment

Using HRCT images visual assessment bronchial wall thickness and the extent of emphysema were the strongest independent determinants of a decreased FEV_1 in patients with mild to extensive emphysema.[33] However, visual assessment of bronchial wall thickening is highly subjective and poorly reproducible.[34] The quantitative analysis can be performed by manual delineation of bronchial contours.[35] Nakano and colleagues[36,37] were the first to perform quantitative measurements of airway wall thickening in COPD patients and reported a significant correlation between wall thickness of the apical right upper lobe bronchus and $FEV_1\%$ predicted. Due to technical limitations of HRCT, neither the generation of the bronchus measured could be determined nor could measurements be performed exactly perpendicular to the axis of the bronchus. It was also demonstrated that the normalized airway wall thickness was larger in smokers with COPD than in smokers or nonsmokers without COPD.[38] Unfortunately, the measurements were restricted to bronchi running almost perpendicular to the transverse CT section. Based on these experiences it is obvious that the complexity and size of the bronchial tree render manual measurement methods impractical and inaccurate.[39]

The dramatically increased acquisition velocity of MSCT, which reduced motion artifacts, and the increasing spatial resolution (especially

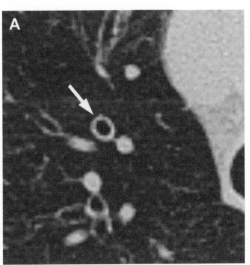

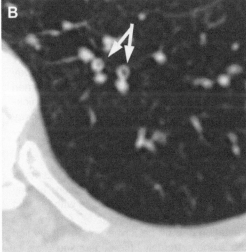

Fig. 3. Mild bronchial dilation without wall thickening (*A, arrow*) and moderate bronchial wall thickening without dilatation (*B, arrow*) of subsegmental bronchi, typical for the airway predominant type of COPD.

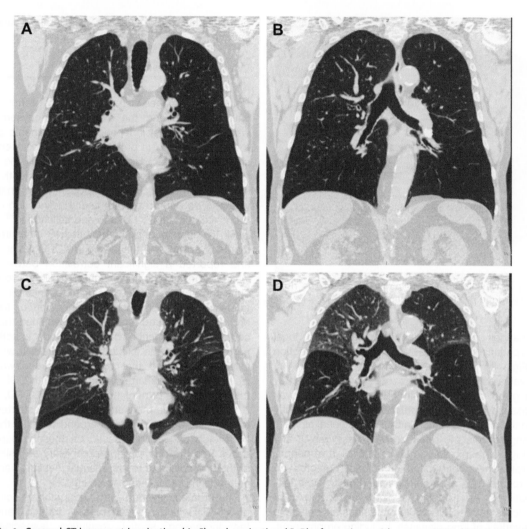

Fig. 4. Coronal CT images at inspiration (*A, B*) and expiration (*C, D*) of a patient with severe COPD (GOLD stage 3) showing massive air trapping of the lower lobes. The upper lobes and middle lobe show a normal increase in density after exhalation.

z-axis-resolution), opened the door to quantitative evaluation of airway dimensions down to subsegmental bronchial level. Volumetric CT allows for quantitative indices of bronchial airway morphology to be calculated, including lumen area, airway inner and outer diameters, wall thicknesses, wall area, airway segment lengths, airway taper indices, and airway branching patterns.

Automatic assessment

The use of curved MPR from 3D-CT datasets is a simple solution to accurately measure airway dimensions regardless of their course with respect to the transaxial CT scan (**Fig. 5**). Airway tree segmentation can be performed manually, which is tedious and extremely time consuming.[40]

On the basis of the volumetric data sets sophisticated post processing tools will automatically segment the airways down to the sixth generation.[8] This allows for visualization of the tracheobronchial tree without any overlap by surrounding parenchyma and for the reproducible and reliable measurements of the segmented airways.

The simplest segmentation method used a single threshold (cutoff) of pixel values in Hounsfield units (HU). Pixels with HU values lower than the threshold were assigned to the lumen (air), while surrounding pixels with HU values higher than the threshold were assigned to the airway wall or other surrounding tissue. Based on this analysis, the 3D region growing algorithm extracts all voxels that are definitely airway. However, using a simple global threshold often fails in detecting the wall of smaller airways; thereby such tools often require manual editing. To enhance this

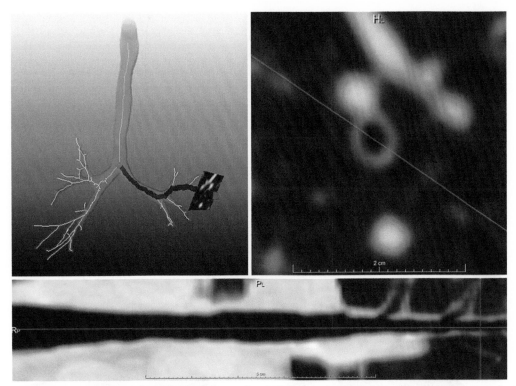

Fig. 5. Volumetric CT datasets allow for 3D segmentation and skeletonization of the airways. In this example, the centerline of the left upper bronchi was used to generate a curved MPR, and subsequently, a perpendicular display of the bronchus. Images were generated using MeVIS software (Bremen, Germany).

basic segmentation process some additional (add-on) algorithms were developed, (ie, based on fuzzy connectivity[41] or by wave propagation from the border voxels).[8] The luminal segmentation result is condensed to the centerline (or skeletization) running exactly in the center of the airway. These centerline points are the starting points for the airway wall detection and quantification. Approaches include methods based on the estimation of the full width at half-maximum (FWHM), brightness-area product and pixel-intensity gradient.[38,41–44] The most frequently reported method is based on the FWHM approach[45] that is explained in more detail; by identifying the lumen center, the scheme measures pixel values along radial rays casting from the lumen center outward beyond the airway wall in all directions. Along each ray, the boundary between the lumen and wall is determined by a pixel whose HU value is half the range between the local minimum in the lumen and the local maximum in the airway wall; while the boundary between the wall and lung parenchyma is determined by a pixel whose HU value is half the range between the local maximum in the wall and the local minimum in the parenchyma. Along each radial ray, these two FWHM

pixels are used as the inner and outer (beginning and ending) pixels of the airway wall. All pixels inside the first FWHM pixel are assigned to a lumen and all pixels outside the second FWHM pixel are assigned to the lung parenchyma. The measurements with the simple FWHM method result in unacceptable large errors for wall thicknesses smaller than 1.0 mm. A new method of integral based closed-form solution based on the volume conservation property of convolution showed precise results.[46] The integral under the profile is kept constant, while the profile itself is transformed, narrowed, and elevated (**Fig. 6**).

Quantitative measurements revealed high correlations between airway luminal area, and to a lesser extent for wall thickening, with $FEV_1\%$ predicted in patients with COPD. The correlation actually improved as airway size decreased from the third ($r = 0.6$ for airway luminal area and $r = 0.43$ for wall thickening) to sixth bronchial generation ($r = 0.73$ and $r = 0.55$, respectively).[47]

By using integral-based method, the mean wall percentage, mean wall thickness, and median wall thickness in nonsmokers (29.6%; 0.69 mm; 0.37 mm) was significantly different ($P<.001$) from the COPD (smokers, GOLD stage 2 and 3) group

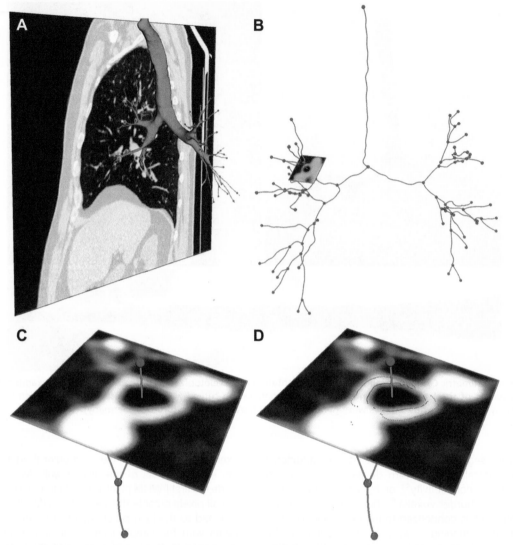

Fig. 6. (*A, B*) 3D-segmentation of the tracheobronchial tree with the centerline (*green line*) and branching points (*red dots*). Automatic segmentation of the inner and outer diameter of the airways is performed on images perpendicular to the centerline (*C, D*). Images were generated using YACTA software (Oliver Weinheimer, University of Mainz, Germany).

(38.9%; 0.83 mm; 0.54 mm). Correlation between FEV_1 and FEV_1 % predicted and the wall percentage for airways greater than 4 mm in diameter was $r = -0.532$ and $r = -0.541$, respectively. Correlation was higher ($r = -0.621$ and $r = -0.537$) when only airways of 4 mm diameter in total and smaller were considered.[48]

Identifying mucoid impacted airways is also important for the clinical practice. For the automatic detection the branch points are extrapolated at each terminal branch along its axis to extract 2D cross-sections that are subsequently matched to a model of mucus plugging computed from the dimensions of the terminal branch.[9] Up until now,

this feature is still experimental; however, first tests have demonstrated promising results.

MAGNETIC RESONANCE IMAGING
Technical Aspects

Overall, the use of MR imaging for assessment of airways is limited. Therefore, mainly our experiences can be provided.

The most frequently used sequences in MR imaging of obstructive lung disease are acquired in a breathhold. For fast T2-weighted imaging, single-shot techniques with partial-Fourier acquisition (HASTE) or ultrashort TE (UTSE) are recommended. The T2-weighted HASTE sequence in coronal or axial orientation allows for the depiction of pulmonary infiltrates, inflammatory bronchial wall thickening and mucus collections. T1-weighted 3D gradient echo sequences, such as VIBE, are suitable for the assessment of the mediastinum and common nodular lesions. The intravenous application of contrast material markedly improves the diagnostic yield of T1-weighted sequences by a clearer depiction of vessels, hilar structures and solid pathologies. A major goal in inflammatory obstructive airway disease is to differentiate inflammation within the wall from muscular hypertrophy, edema, and mucus collection which cannot be achieved by CT, but can be addressed by the use of T1- and T2-weighted images and contrast enhancement.

Qualitative Evaluation

Trachea

The depiction of airway dimensions and size of the airway walls by MR imaging under physiologic conditions is limited to the central bronchi. In the authors own experience, the trachea can be best visualized by a T1w 3D volume interpolated gradient echo sequence (VIBE). For perception of TBM, MR imaging should be acquired in inspiratory and expiratory breath hold. For dynamic assessment of tracheal instability MR cine acquisitions during continuous respiration or forced expiration are recommended.[24] For data acquisition, time resolved techniques are used which can be based on FLASH or trueFISP sequences. This allows for a high temporal resolution down to 100 ms per frame.

Large airways

For depiction of the bronchiectasis high spatial resolution is essential (Fig. 7). By using a 3D volume interpolated gradient echo sequence (VIBE) with a voxel size of approximately 0.9 × 0.88 × 2.5 mm^3 a sensitivity of 79% and a specificity of 98% regarding the visual depiction of bronchiectasis was shown compared with CT.[49]

Functional Imaging

The major advantage of MR imaging is the functional imaging. Ventilation and perfusion can be directly visualized by MR imaging. Several different techniques are available, with oxygen enhancement and inhalation of hyperpolarized noble gases being the most prominent. Oxygen-enhanced MR imaging requires no special scanner hardware, is easy to use, and the costs for oxygen are low. However, the use of high oxygen

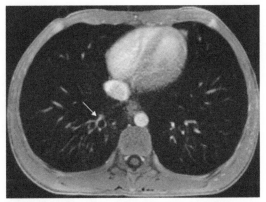

Fig. 7. MR imaging (axial T1-weighted GE sequence post contrast [VIBE]) showing severe bronchial dilatation especially of the right lower lobe (*arrows*).

concentrations (15 L/min) may be risky in patients with severe COPD. ^{3}Helium MR imaging is based on the inhalation of hyperpolarized ^{3}helium gas. It allows for direct evaluation of the distribution of the tracer gas after a breath hold (static) or during continuous breathing (dynamic) and airspace dimensions. The latter is done by diffusion-weighted MR imaging. Areas with ventilation defects caused by airway obstruction and emphysema represent the only limitation because they cannot be assessed due to lack of the tracer gas entering these areas. Thus, there is almost no information about these affected lung regions. Overall, the high cost of the noble gas ^{3}helium, the process of laser-induced hyperpolarization, and the need for nonproton imaging remain the major drawbacks of this technology on its way to broader clinical applications.

Due to the reflex of hypoxic vasoconstriction, ventilation defects in COPD largely correspond to perfusion defects in the same areas. Thus, the assessment of pulmonary perfusion makes a lot of sense, especially as perfusion MR imaging is much easier and more straightforward than ventilation MR imaging. The basic principle of contrast-enhanced perfusion MR imaging is a dynamic acquisition during and after an intravenous bolus injection of a paramagnetic contrast agent. Perfusion MR imaging of the lung requires a high-temporal resolution to visualize the peak enhancement of the lung parenchyma. Consequently, contrast-enhanced perfusion MR imaging uses T1-weighted gradient echo MR imaging with ultra-short TR and TE, such as FLASH. With the introduction of parallel imaging techniques, 3D perfusion imaging, with a high spatial and temporal resolution and an improved anatomic coverage and z-axis resolution, can be acquired.[50–52] These data sets are also well suited

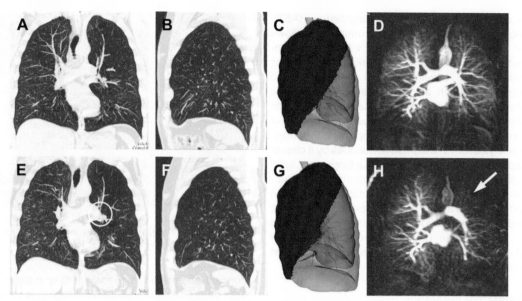

Fig. 8. Coronal and sagittal images (5 mm MIP) in a patient with severe emphysema: initial examination (*A–D*) and 6 months after the placement of the endobrochial valves (*circle*) in the left upper lobe (*E–H*). The interlobar fissure moved slightly upwards after the therapy suggesting a volume reduction of the left upper lobe. By quantitative measurement the volume of the treated lung can be assessed, but only a small shift of volume from the left upper to the lower lobe was found (the volume of the left lung remains the same while the volume of the upper lobe decreased by 300 mL). The corresponding MR perfusion (50 mm MIP images) shows hypoxic vasoconstriction in the left upper lobe (*arrow*) with redistribution of perfusion to ventilated areas. This example demonstrates nicely the small volume difference after therapy but with a significant functional change.

for high quality multiplanar reformats. Due to high spatial resolution, detailed analysis of pulmonary perfusion and precise anatomic localization of the perfusion defects on a lobar, and even segmental level, can be performed. By applying the principles of indicator dilution techniques perfusion MR imaging allows for the quantitative evaluation of pulmonary blood volume and flow. The influence of ventilation on perfusion is nicely illustrated in Fig. 8, where a patient undergoing endobronchial valve placement only shows a minor volume decrease of the treated lung, whereas perfusion is shifted away from the treated part of the lung to the other parts which are then better perfused.

SUMMARY

Visualization of airways in COPD patients is important for understanding the disease and therapeutic management. Today a 3D HRCT dataset is recommended, allowing for perpendicular visualization and measurements of airways diameter and wall thickness. Modern postprocessing software allows for automatic segmentation and quantification. Additional expiratory scans demonstrate the extent of central tracheobronchomalacia and peripheral small airway obstruction. MR imaging

is well suited for dynamic assessment of tracheal instability and for gaining functional information on perfusion and ventilation in COPD.

REFERENCES

1. GOLD Global strategy for the diagnosis, management, and prevention of chronic obstructive pulmonary disease. Executive summary, updated November 2008. Available at: http://www.gold copd.org.
2. Snider G, Kleinerman J, Thurlbeck WM, et al. The definition of emphysema. Report of a national heart, lung, and blood institute, division of lung diseases workshop. Am Rev Respir Dis 1985;132:182–5.
3. Hogg JC, Chu F, Utokaparch S, et al. The nature of small-airway obstruction in chronic obstructive pulmonary disease. N Engl J Med 2004;350: 2645–53.
4. Hogg JC. State of the art. Bronchiolitis in chronic obstructive pulmonary disease. Proc Am Thorac Soc 2006;3:489–93.
5. Mayo JR. MR imaging of pulmonary parenchyma. Magn Reson Imaging Clin N Am 2000;8:105–23.
6. Ley-Zaporozhan J, Ley S, Kauczor HU. Proton MRI in COPD. COPD 2007;4:55–65.
7. Goldin JG. Quantitative CT of the lung. Radiol Clin North Am 2002;40:145–62.

8. Mayer D, Bartz D, Fischer J, et al. Hybrid segmentation and virtual bronchoscopy based on CT images. Acad Radiol 2004;11:551–65.

9. Kiraly AP, Odry BL, Godoy MC, et al. Computer-aided diagnosis of the airways: beyond nodule detection. J Thorac Imaging 2008;23:105–13.

10. Grenier PA, Beigelman-Aubry C, Fetita C, et al. Multidetector-row CT of the airways. Semin Roentgenol 2003;38:146–57.

11. Fetita CI, Preteux F, Beigelman-Aubry C, et al. Pulmonary airways: 3-D reconstruction from multislice CT and clinical investigation. IEEE Trans Med Imaging 2004;23:1353–64.

12. Grenier PA, Beigelman-Aubry C, Fetita C, et al. New frontiers in CT imaging of airway disease. Eur Radiol 2002;12:1022–44.

13. Lee YK, Oh YM, Lee JH, et al. Quantitative assessment of emphysema, air trapping, and airway thickening on computed tomography. Lung 2008;186:157–65.

14. Beigelman-Aubry C, Hill C, Guibal A, et al. Multidetector row CT and postprocessing techniques in the assessment of diffuse lung disease. Radiographics 2005;25:1639–52.

15. Zompatori M, Battaglia M, Rimondi MR, et al. [Quantitative assessment of pulmonary emphysema with computerized tomography. Comparison of the visual score and high resolution computerized tomography, expiratory density mask with spiral computerized tomography and respiratory function tests]. Radiol Med 1997;93:374–81 [in Italian].

16. Brillet PY, Fetita CI, Saragaglia A, et al. Investigation of airways using MDCT for visual and quantitative assessment in COPD patients. Int J Chron Obstruct Pulmon Dis 2008;3:97–107.

17. Kauczor HU, Wolcke B, Fischer B, et al. Three-dimensional helical CT of the tracheobronchial tree: evaluation of imaging protocols and assessment of suspected stenoses with bronchoscopic correlation. AJR Am J Roentgenol 1996;167:419–24.

18. Zhang J, Hasegawa I, Feller-Kopman D, et al. 2003 AUR memorial award. Dynamic expiratory volumetric CT imaging of the central airways: comparison of standard-dose and low-dose techniques. Acad Radiol 2003;10:719–24.

19. Verschakelen JA, Scheinbaum K, Bogaert J, et al. Expiratory CT in cigarette smokers: correlation between areas of decreased lung attenuation, pulmonary function tests and smoking history. Eur Radiol 1998;8:1391–9.

20. Kauczor HU, Hast J, Heussel CP, et al. Focal airtrapping at expiratory high-resolution CT: comparison with pulmonary function tests. Eur Radiol 2000;10:1539–46.

21. Hansell DM. Small airways diseases: detection and insights with computed tomography. Eur Respir J 2001;17:1294–313.

22. Loring SH, O'Donnell CR, Feller-Kopman DJ, et al. Central airway mechanics and flow limitation in acquired tracheobronchomalacia. Chest 2007;131:1118–24.

23. Jokinen K, Palva T, Nuutinen J. Chronic bronchitis. A bronchologic evaluation. ORL J Otorhinolaryngol Relat Spec 1976;38:178–86.

24. Heussel CP, Ley S, Biedermann A, et al. Respiratory lumenal change of the pharynx and trachea in normal subjects and COPD patients: assessment by cine-MRI. Eur Radiol 2004;14:2188–97.

25. Boiselle PM, Ernst A. Tracheal morphology in patients with tracheomalacia: prevalence of inspiratory lunate and expiratory "frown" shapes. J Thorac Imaging 2006;21:190–6.

26. Kim SJ, Im JG, Kim IO, et al. Normal bronchial and pulmonary arterial diameters measured by thin section CT. J Comput Assist Tomogr 1995;19:365–9.

27. Kim JS, Muller NL, Park CS, et al. Bronchoarterial ratio on thin section CT: comparison between high altitude and sea level. J Comput Assist Tomogr 1997;21:306–11.

28. Imaging of disease of the chest. In: Hansell DM, Armstrong P, Lynch DA, et al, editors. 4th edition. London: Elsevier Mosby 2005.

29. Webb WR. Thin-section CT of the secondary pulmonary lobule: anatomy and the image–the 2004 Fleischner lecture. Radiology 2006;239:322–38.

30. Zaporozhan J, Ley S, Eberhardt R, et al. Paired inspiratory/expiratory volumetric thin-slice CT scan for emphysema analysis: comparison of different quantitative evaluations and pulmonary function test. Chest 2005;128:3212–20.

31. Baldi S, Miniati M, Bellina CR, et al. Relationship between extent of pulmonary emphysema by high-resolution computed tomography and lung elastic recoil in patients with chronic obstructive pulmonary disease. Am J Respir Crit Care Med 2001;164:585–9.

32. Berger P, Laurent F, Begueret H, et al. Structure and function of small airways in smokers: relationship between air trapping at CT and airway inflammation. Radiology 2003;228:85–94.

33. Aziz ZA, Wells AU, Desai SR, et al. Functional impairment in emphysema: contribution of airway abnormalities and distribution of parenchymal disease. AJR Am J Roentgenol 2005;185:1509–15.

34. Park JW, Hong YK, Kim CW, et al. High-resolution computed tomography in patients with bronchial asthma: correlation with clinical features, pulmonary functions and bronchial hyperresponsiveness. J Investig Allergol Clin Immunol 1997;7:186–92.

35. Orlandi I, Moroni C, Camiciottoli G, et al. Chronic obstructive pulmonary disease: thin-section CT measurement of airway wall thickness and lung attenuation. Radiology 2005;234:604–10.

36. Nakano Y, Muro S, Sakai H, et al. Computed tomographic measurements of airway dimensions and emphysema in smokers. Correlation with lung function. Am J Respir Crit Care Med 2000;162:1102–8.

37. Nakano Y, Muller NL, King GG, et al. Quantitative assessment of airway remodeling using high-resolution CT. Chest 2002;122:271S–5S.

38. Berger P, Perot V, Desbarats P, et al. Airway wall thickness in cigarette smokers: quantitative thin-section CT assessment. Radiology 2005;235: 1055–64.

39. Venkatraman R, Raman R, Raman B, et al. Fully automated system for three-dimensional bronchial morphology analysis using volumetric multidetector computed tomography of the chest. J Digit Imaging 2006;19:132–9.

40. Aykac D, Hoffman EA, McLennan G, et al. Segmentation and analysis of the human airway tree from three-dimensional X-ray CT images. IEEE Trans Med Imaging 2003;22:940–50.

41. Tschirren J, Hoffman EA, McLennan G, et al. Segmentation and quantitative analysis of intrathoracic airway trees from computed tomography images. Proc Am Thorac Soc 2005;2:484–7 503–484.

42. Reinhardt JM, D'Souza ND, Hoffman EA. Accurate measurement of intrathoracic airways. IEEE Trans Med Imaging 1997;16:820–7.

43. Saba OI, Hoffman EA, Reinhardt JM. Maximizing quantitative accuracy of lung airway lumen and wall measures obtained from X-ray CT imaging. J Appl Phys 2003;95:1063–75.

44. Nakano Y, Wong JC, de Jong PA, et al. The prediction of small airway dimensions using computed tomography. Am J Respir Crit Care Med 2005;171: 142–6.

45. de Jong PA, Muller NL, Pare PD, et al. Computed tomographic imaging of the airways: relationship to structure and function. Eur Respir J 2005;26: 140–52.

46. Weinheimer O, Achenbach T, Bletz C, et al. About objective 3-d analysis of airway geometry in computerized tomography. IEEE Trans Med Imaging 2008;27:64–74.

47. Hasegawa M, Nasuhara Y, Onodera Y, et al. Airflow limitation and airway dimensions in chronic obstructive pulmonary disease. Am J Respir Crit Care Med 2006;173:1309–15.

48. Achenbach T, Weinheimer O, Biedermann A, et al. MDCT assessment of airway wall thickness in COPD patients using a new method: correlations with pulmonary function tests. Eur Radiol 2008; 18(12):2731–8.

49. Biederer J, Both M, Graessner J, et al. Lung morphology: fast MR imaging assessment with a volumetric interpolated breath-hold technique: initial experience with patients. Radiology 2003; 226:242–9.

50. Ley S, Fink C, Puderbach M, et al. Contrast-enhanced 3D MR perfusion of the lung: application of parallel imaging technique in healthy subjects. Rofo 2004;176:330–4.

51. Fink C, Puderbach M, Bock M, et al. Regional lung perfusion: assessment with partially parallel three-dimensional MR imaging. Radiology 2004;231: 175–84.

52. Fink C, Ley S, Kroeker R, et al. Time-resolved contrast-enhanced three-dimensional magnetic resonance angiography of the chest: combination of parallel imaging with view sharing (TREAT). Invest Radiol 2005;40:40–8.

Index

Note: Page numbers of article titles are in **boldface** type.

Radiol Clin N Am 47 (2009) 343–347
doi:10.1016/S0033-8389(09)00042-6

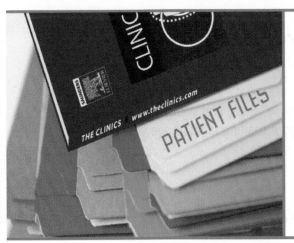
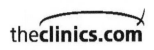

Moving?

Make sure your subscription moves with you!

To notify us of your new address, find your **Clinics Account Number** (located on your mailing label above your name), and contact customer service at:

E-mail: elspcs@elsevier.com

800-654-2452 (subscribers in the U.S. & Canada)
314-453-7041 (subscribers outside of the U.S. & Canada)

Fax number: 314-523-5170

Elsevier Periodicals Customer Service
11830 Westline Industrial Drive
St. Louis, MO 63146

*To ensure uninterrupted delivery of your subscription, please notify us at least 4 weeks in advance of move.

Printed and bound by CPI Group (UK) Ltd, Croydon, CR0 4YY

03/10/2024

01040355-0014